GN00818598

SPORTS NUTRITION
IN PRACTICE

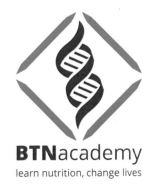

BTNacademy

learn nutrition, change lives

Self-published by The BTN Academy, a trading name of Ben Coomber Ltd

First edition, October 2018

Copyright 2018

The moral right of Ben Coomber Ltd to be identified as the author of this work has been asserted in accordance with the Copyright, Designs and Patents Act, 1988.

All rights reserved. No part of this publication may be reproduced or transmitted in any form or by any means, electronic or mechanical, without the prior permission of the author, Ben Coomber, or Ben Coomber Ltd.

ISBN: 978-1-9996560-2-7

Written by Tom Bainbridge, Ben Coomber, Dave Crosland and Phil Paterson

Designed by Charlotte Thompson

Edited by Charlotte Thompson and Tom Bainbridge

Book cover designed by Holly Brookes

Dedication

Our mission as a company is allow you, the student, to learn nutrition that changes lives. If we teach you these life skills we have a meaningful impact on the world, and for us that is a mission worth working hard for.

Thus, this book is dedicated to you, our students, because without your hard work and effort we would not be able to achieve what we have set out to do. With this book acting as your guide, it is our hope that you will be able to go on to help hundreds if not thousands of other people improve their health, body composition and overall wellbeing. After all nutrition is a life skill but without people like you many will never develop it and realise their true health potential.

You make our mission possible, thank you.

Table of contents

INTRODUCTION 8

HOW TO USE THIS MANUAL 9

22. MODULE 22: EVIDENCE-BASED NUTRITION FOR ENDURANCE SPORT 11

    22.1. Module aims 11

    22.2. Key principles from module 21 11

    22.3. Introduction to evidence-based nutrition for endurance sport 11

    22.4. Calorie calculation and energy requirements for endurance athletes 12

    22.5. Energy balancing 13

    22.6. Summarising athlete weight management 15

    22.7. Macronutrient balancing for endurance athletes 15

    22.8. Protein intake for endurance athletes 16

    22.9. Nutrition periodisation 18

    22.10. Energy systems and muscle fibre type 19

    22.11. Ketogenic diets and endurance performance 22

    22.12. Fasted training for endurance performance 23

    22.13. Metabolic flexibility and insulin resistance 23

    22.14. Race week, the taper and carbohydrate (CHO) loading 24

    22.15. Caution with carbohydrate loading 26

    22.16. Modern adaptations 26

    22.17. How much is enough? 27

    22.18. Estimated energy stores in humans 27

    22.19. Race day nutrition 28

    22.20. In-race fuelling 28

    22.21. Carbohydrate types and gastric emptying rates 30

    22.22. Logistics in-race fuelling and examples 30

    22.23. Race day supplementation 32

    22.24. Relative Energy Deficiency in Sport (RED-S) 32

    22.25. Health consequences of RED-S 33

    22.26. Summary 33

    22.27. References 35

Table of contents

23. MODULE 23: ASSISTED ATHLETES **40**

    23.1.   Module aims 40

    23.2.   Key principles from module 22 40

    23.3.   Introduction to assisted athletes 40

    23.4.   What are steroids? 41

    23.5.   The business of steroids 44

    23.6.   IPED users 45

        23.6.1.   Competitive bodybuilders/strength sports 45

        23.6.2.   Aspiring competitors 46

        23.6.3.   Image users 46

        23.6.4.   Sports athletes 47

        23.6.5.   Therapeutic users 47

        23.6.6.   Fat loss group 47

        23.6.7.   Armed and emergency services 47

    23.7.   How steroids are used 48

        23.7.1.   Periodic cycle 48

        23.7.2.   Blast/cruise 48

    23.8.   Hormone Replacement Therapy (HRT) 48

    23.9.   Natural hormone production 50

    23.10. Post-Cycle Therapy (PCT) 51

    23.11. Physical harms 53

        23.11.1. Infertility 53

        23.11.2. Cardiac 54

        23.11.3. Renal issues 54

        23.11.4. Liver incidents 54

        23.11.5. Muscular and tendon injury 54

        23.11.6. Blood Born Viruses (BBV) 55

        23.11.7. Hypothyroidism 55

        23.11.8. Mental health 55

    23.12. The current situation with IPEDS within the UK today 56

Table of contents

23.13. Drug availability.. 57

23.14. Do we know just how much Is out there?..................................... 57

23.15. The driving forces?.. 58

23.16. How do the drugs differ? 61

23.17. What are the most common drugs 65

23.18. Selective Androgen Receptor Modulators (SARMS) 67

23.19. Summary 68

23.20. References 71

24. MODULE 24: TEAM SPORTS NUTRITION **73**

24.1. Module aims 73

24.2. Key principles from module 23 73

24.3. Introduction to team sports nutrition 73

24.4. Build a Foundation 74

24.5. Macronutrient intake 76

24.6. Building good habits... 78

24.7. Setting up the week 79

24.8. Game day considerations... 80

24.9. Recovery tactics after games 81

24.10. Season timing and other considerations.................................. 83

24.11. Body composition improvements as an athlete (2) 83

24.12. Fat loss with an athlete 84

24.13. Weight gain with an athlete.. 85

24.14. Coaching a team/club 85

24.15. Summary 87

24.16. References 88

25. MODULE 25: NUTRITION FOR BODYBUILDING PREP **90**

25.1. Module aims 90

25.2. Key principles from module 24 90

25.3. Introduction to nutrition for bodybuilding prep 90

25.4. What is contest prep? 92

Table of contents

25.5.   How lean are we talking? 93

25.6.   When are you ready? 94

25.7.   Prep: The basics 95

25.8.   Calories 96

25.9.   Macronutrient recommendations for contest prep 98

25.10. Peak week nutrition 103

25.11. Training during prep 105

25.12. Health consequences of prep 106

25.13. Post-show nutrition and rebounding 108

25.14. Summary 110

25.15. References 112

26.   MODULE 26: NUTRITIONAL CONSIDERATIONS FOR MAKING WEIGHT 115

26.1.   Module aims 115

26.2.   Key principles from module 25 115

26.3.   Introduction to nutritional considerations for making weight 116

26.4.   What are the weight classes? 116

26.5.   What is making weight? 118

26.6.   Choosing a weight category 121

26.7.   Choosing a weight category based on body fat level 122

26.8.   Losing weight 122

26.9.   Weigh-in times 124

26.10. Depletion phase 125

26.11. Refuelling and hydration strategies 128

26.12. Summary and off-season weight 130

26.13. References 131

INTRODUCTION

Welcome to Sports Nutrition in Practice, a practical nutrition coaching manual for aspiring sports nutritionists.

Nutrition as a topic is far more vast than the simple promotion of good health and/or body composition. Because at some basic level food really is just fuel, the choices we make at the dinner table can have a profound effect on our performance in the gym, on the pitch, and any other athletic environment. While it may be the case that performance – even peak performance – can be achieved with a less than optimal diet (as evidenced by the eating habits of many top athletes) it is still the case that when all else is equal an athlete will get better results if a few key nutritional principles are adhered to. After all, sports nutrition has come a long way since the 80's, where the advice was little more than "Eat as much carbohydrate as possible and stay hydrated".

This book seeks to build upon The Art of Nutrition Coaching by showing you the means by which key nutrition principles, and the artful application of them, can apply specifically to those in a competitive athletic environment. The latter point is critical here and so while you read this book it's important to bear in mind all you have learned about environmental cues, motivation, readiness to change and proper communicative techniques. We must never forget that athletes are people, too, with all of the same barriers to success. This means that while you may expect an athlete to adhere to whatever nutritional approach you recommend without question, you'll quickly learn while working in this space that your assumption is incorrect.

Here we will cover various different sporting populations, specifically endurance athletes, team sport athletes, athletes that need to make weight for competition, and athletes preparing for a physique competition. We will also look in to the world of IPED use to help you become more informed and aware should a client ever bring the topic up with you.

While reading this book, keep in mind that each sport is chosen not only to illustrate itself, but also a wider principle. The information about training endurance sports, for example, can be used with footballers, or combined with what you already know about supporting muscle growth and recovery before being applied to Crossfit athletes or boxers who aren't currently in preparation for a fight. This book may be relatively short, but in combination with the previous BTN Academy modules and manuals you have a handbook for working with just about any athlete of any discipline.

Time to find out what makes an athlete tick.

Tom Bainbridge and Ben Coomber

HOW TO USE THIS MANUAL

This book will take on the following structure:

- **Module 22:** Evidence-based nutrition for endurance sport

- **Module 23:** Assisted athletes

- **Module 24:** Team sports nutrition

- **Module 25:** Nutrition for bodybuilding prep

- **Module 26:** Nutritional considerations for making weight

Each module in this book can be read as a stand-alone lesson, but when accompanying the BTN Practical Academy, it will act as your course reading material and is to be considered pre-reading before viewing each module's video. This is our teaching mantra, read, watch, discuss and apply, re-reading and re-watching until the modules are mastered and applicability is understood. This approach gives you the best chance to absorb as much information as possible without spending hours at your desk unnecessarily, all while setting you up to maximise your understanding of any given topic.

We hope you enjoy this book, as it's time to learn…

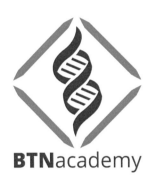

BTNacademy

MODULE 22

EVIDENCE-BASED NUTRITION FOR ENDURANCE SPORT

22.   MODULE 22: EVIDENCE-BASED NUTRITION FOR ENDURANCE SPORT

22.1. Module aims

- Understand how to properly fuel an endurance athlete and assist them in maintaining weight during different phases of training and competition

- Learn about specific nutritional protocols for ensuring athletes are able to perform at their best, including immune system function, hydration and event fuelling

- Appreciate nutrition periodisation; what is it and how to use it for your athletes

- Understand why ketogenic dieting might not be not optimal for endurance athletes despite its recent popularity

- Investigate the benefits of fasted cardio for the endurance athlete

- To give students an appreciation for how carbohydrate manipulation, if done right, can improve performance and to become familiar with Carbohydrate (CHO) loading protocols

- To explain the protocol for 'race week'

- Students will understand the impact of sports nutrition on endurance performance

22.2. Key principles from module 21

In the last module we covered alcoholic drinks and their effect on body composition, health, calorie intake and broader behaviour. You learned:

- Alcohol research is difficult to parse out, being predominantly based in epidemiology which has inherent flaws that are difficult to impossible to overcome

- Alcohol calories influence overall balance in a very similar way to carbohydrate and so should be considered

- Most alcoholic drinks have carbohydrate calories alongside alcohol, meaning the calories stack up faster than you'd expect

- Alcohol negatively affects sleep, choices around food and overall energy the following day (which can also then negatively affect behaviour)

- Moderate drinking (defined as less than 10 units per week) is likely to be benign as part of a healthy lifestyle

- Moderate drinking is often reported to reduce risk compared to being teetotal. As based on epidemiology, this 'fact' is not above criticism and so it is not an evidence-based position to encourage those that do not drink to take up the habit

22.3. Introduction to evidence-based nutrition for endurance sport

In its simplest form, fuelling any athlete is about meeting their calorie and nutrient demands so they can train effectively, recover fully, and maintain optimal health. Therefore, in order to meet the demands of your athlete, it's important that we understand the demands of their sport(s) and the energy systems that will be utilised during training and competition. By doing this we will be able to account for everything they need.

Understanding your client's goals is an important first step in working out what kind of nutrition strategy you are going to implement. In some respects, training a full-time or elite athlete is easier than your amateur athlete or weekend warrior since, not only are their day to day training and lifestyle routines more predictable and easier to manage, their level of commitment and adherence is typically higher. However, for most of us, it's about balancing training with work and life commitments. It's important that you establish what your client or athlete's goals are, so you can be sure that they are realistic and don't clash with each other. For example, body image and performance goals don't always go hand in hand because one of them relies on a calorie deficit (or at least avoidance of a surplus) while the other, in most cases, should be approached by erring on the side of overeating rather than risking not eating enough when in doubt.

Trying to get your clients to focus on the nutrient value of their food first from a recovery and performance perspective, means they'll focus on the positive aspects of eating and how it can make them feel good. With the fitness industry being very image focused it can be easy to forget that training and eating are about making us feel and perform better, not just look better. Encourage your clients and athletes to train to perform and eat to fuel performance. Nowhere is this truer than in the world of endurance sports where energy requirements tend to be higher than in any other discipline. Proper fuelling may involve taking on thousands of calories more than are needed by individuals partaking in other sports, and so an athlete scared to eat lest they gain fat is going to struggle to recover and improve over time.

As well as meeting the demands of day to day training and of competing, we also need to address the logistics of taking on nutrition during an event. As such, in this module we will cover the basics, before looking at two examples within multi-sport of how modern fuelling strategies have evolved.

22.4. Calorie calculation and energy requirements for endurance athletes

As you have already learned in an earlier module, calculating Basal Metabolic Rate (BMR) and Total Daily Energy Expenditure (TDEE) can be done using the Harris-Benedict equation. This will provide you with a baseline, a starting point. An alternative starting point might well be the information provided through a food diary. Providing the tracking is accurate and you can coach your athlete into a state of consistency, you can see how many calories they consume on average and if their current weight isn't fluctuating, then you will have a fairly accurate TDEE. There are pros and cons of both methods, and one option might be to calculate BMR and TDEE using both methods and split the difference. We tend to recommend simply using an equation to estimate and then going by trial and error; you have already learned about the fallibility of self-reported nutritional intakes!

A question that is raised at this point is: "Why do precise nutrient requirements need to be calculated at all?". Surely an athlete knows they need to eat more before and after training, and less on days they don't train. They also need to eat a lot before competition, so why bother with the precision? The problem with a looser approach is twofold:

- Those prone to overeating will gain unwanted weight

- Those prone to undereating will under eat, resulting in impaired recovery and subsequent performance

In many endurance sports, performance can be improved with a better power to weight ratio (meaning your ability to generate force compared to your bodyweight. In theory if two athletes can produce X force, the lighter athlete will be able to move faster). This is true in cycling where a lighter athlete will be able to accelerate and climb more effectively. While training will increase strength and power, for many athletes, especially towards the amateur end of the scale, the most effective way to improve power to weight ratio may mean dropping bodyweight. In runners, a reduced bodyweight can also reduce the ground reaction force upon foot-strike, therefore reducing energy demands and the amount of impact stress on the body, which may reduce the risk of injury too. Because of this it's important to maintain a certain weight at which the athlete does not feel heavy, but at the same time we cannot risk undereating when trying to stay light. Precision is therefore important.

If an athlete is too heavy at present and genuinely does need to lose some fat, they must be made aware that any weight loss strategies they employ could have negative effects on performance, at least initially, since reduced energy intake may limit training. During periods of increased training volume and intensity e.g. during a build or race phase, any calorie restriction could result in a drop in performance or even increase injury risk if your athlete isn't sufficiently recovered. For this reason, try to keep any weight loss the target of off-season or early season training. It's also prudent to keep calorie deficits small to allow a more gradual weight loss to ensure training quality does not suffer.

For athletes close to their goal weight/race weight already, your focus should be on energy balancing; helping a client perform and recover while avoiding weight gain.

22.5.   Energy balancing

If BMR and TDEE (through exercise) were consistent day to day, maintaining an energy balance would be simple. Indeed, it's relatively simple for most gymgoers because the average gym session doesn't burn **that** many calories and so needs stay similar day to day. However, training for most sports will vary from day to day depending on the focus of that session. Endurance athletes such as marathon runners or cyclists' training will include long endurance sessions of multiple hours, shorter interval type sessions, short speed work sessions as well as strength and conditioning. If we look at multi-sport athletes who may be training for two or three sports, then their training over a four week block might never see two days with exactly the same energy demand. What is the most effective method of maintaining an energy balance when the expenditure is so varied?

There are two ways you might go about this; firstly, having worked out target energy intake for an athlete's day to day activity (without training) you can link their sports watch to MyFitnessPal so that when they train, it assigns more calories to their daily intake allowance.

This method allows athletes to see the effect and energy demands of different sports and session types. It also means the energy replacement is soon after the expenditure so they're less likely to under feed following training. However, the disadvantage of this method is that some athletes might see their energy demands vary wildly from easier days to epic long endurance days, so their intake can vary by as much as 4,000kcal. Some athletes may struggle to consume this much extra food in over one day. Additionally, these watches are not always as accurate as they could be and are completely incapable of tracking calorie burn for any interval or resistance-based training.

The second method is to average out your athlete's training week or month in terms of expected energy expenditure and spread the intake more evenly over the whole week, either with exactly the same daily intake or marginal differences on the higher and lower days. The biggest advantage here is that it's much more manageable and consistent to control portion sizes and appetite. Also, consider that recovery doesn't stop at midnight. Growth and repair are ongoing processes within the body. Spreading the intake more evenly over the week may actually improve energy levels and aid recovery more, and so for numerous reasons this is the method we recommend.

> **Note:** it's worth taking into consideration net vs. gross calorie expenditure when looking at what a sports watch or piece of cardio equipment says regarding energy usage. In short, the calories your watch says you burned include the calories you would have burned anyway if you were not exercising. This means that if your watch says you burned 600kcal, you didn't burn 600kcal more than you would have in that period if you weren't training, you burned that in total. Allow us to explain...

When you calculate a client's BMR you have calculated the energy they will use over 24 hours without exercise or activity in general. If that figure comes out to 1800kcals, for example, they will burn (1800/24=) 75kcal per hour. When you then use their BMR to calculate TDEE you may add, for illustration, 600kcal based upon their activity levels. That 600kcal is not used over 24 hours, however, it's burned over the 16 that they are awake. Dividing the additional calories by waking hours and adding to BMR calorie per hour allows us to see the number of calories a person is likely to use while awake. In this example:

- BMR = 1800kcal/24 = 75 per hour

- Activity = 600kcal/16 = 37.5 per hour

- 75+37.5 = 112.5kcal per hour before training

We can round this to 115kcal. Now if your client's watch tells them that they burned 600kcal in an hour of running, the additional burn is actually only 485. If your clients are then adding an additional 600kcal their diet, they may be over consuming. This difference might not sound like much, but over a 3-4 hour training session, over weeks and months of training, it could mount up quickly. This needs to be considered and so an athlete using a watch to calculate their needs should be made aware of the difference.

To finish off this section we will answer the question "what if my client doesn't have a sports watch?". While this situation is workable it is not ideal, and so we will say up front that the best strategy would simply be to invest in one. Any endurance athlete looking to maximise performance will benefit massively from having some sort of fitness tracker that allows them to track heart rate and energy expenditure. Being that a good quality one will cost less than £100 (the amount most will be spending on trainers) it can be considered a small investment for something that is close to a necessity for precise nutritional planning.

If this situation does arise, however, the only method that can realistically be employed utilises some amount of guesswork. It is generally accepted that running a mile on relatively flat terrain burns somewhere in the region of 80-100kcal (net) depending on athlete weight and cycling the same distance burns roughly half of that. Taking these figures, applying them to your client's training and closely monitoring weight gain and loss can, over time, get you relatively close to their true requirements.

22.6.   Summarising athlete weight management

Athlete weight management involves two different calculations – the calculation of their day to day needs without training, and the calculation of their training requirements. To do this one would calculate their needs for their day to day activity and any strength and conditioning using the methods outlined in earlier modules, then use either a fitness tracker or a close estimate to work out their additional needs.

The athlete would then choose to replace their calorie burn on a day to day basis or on an averaged-out basis across the week or month. The former is arguably easier to calculate while the latter is easier to do. The method chosen is down to the athlete and the effects will be more or less the same, but whatever is chosen the importance cannot be overstated – helping a client properly match their energy needs will improve:

- Health, immune function, bone and reproductive health, and recovery from training

- Ability to meet weight categories in sports such as rowing, boxing, or sailing (crew)

- Aesthetics for gymnastics, synchronised swimming, or physique modelling

- Power to weight ratios in cycling, running, rowing

22.7.   Macronutrient balancing for endurance athletes

Finding the correct macronutrient ratio for your endurance athletes is important to ensure optimal fuelling and recovery of training. This has been known for a long time, and probably one of the most well-known recommendations comes from the GSK (Glaxo-Smith Kline) Human Performance Lab who advise endurance athletes to use a macro-ratio: 15:25:60 (protein, fats, carbohydrate) as a starting point. One issue with macronutrient ratios is that the amounts that they refer to will depend on the total energy intake, which may differ from athlete to athlete depending in their bodies and training goals. For this reason, we cannot take one uniform ratio and apply it to all athletes, or even the same athlete on different days.

Looking back to the previous section, an athlete may consume 2000kcal on a rest day, 2400kcal on an interval day and 3500kcal on a long run day, meaning their protein intake would differ from day to day despite overall needs being not too dissimilar, in that protein synthesis needs don't stop at midnight. We can do better than this blanket recommendation.

How we manipulate macronutrient intake to meet our clients' and athletes' requirements may take some trial and error, but there is a process that can be used across the board. A good place to start, is by ensuring adequate daily protein intake. Since muscle protein synthesis is a constant process, it's important that intake be evenly distributed throughout the day and week. Once this is considered, ensuring a fat intake minimum of around 1 g/kg/bw will mean that immune function is supported. From here the athlete's carbohydrate intake will be determined by overall calorie needs for the particular day in question.

You may wish to keep protein and fats stable throughout the week, then manipulate carbohydrate and calorie intake around different training days to meet the fuelling requirements of those sessions. Alternatively, you may find athletes adhere better to a more even food intake over the week with some slight increases in carbohydrate and caloric intake occurring around higher volume training sessions. In the coming sections we will show you how to apply this in more detail and hopefully help you understand why the recommendations are as they are.

22.8. Protein intake for endurance athletes

Increased protein intake and supplementation has long been a part of resistance training and power sports nutrition, with these athletes often consuming more than their endurance focused counterparts. However, it's a mistake to think that endurance athletes do not need to pay attention to this area. While sedentary individuals may meet their dietary requirements for protein intake with around 1.4g/kg/bw or even less, needs for athletes may be considerably higher (1).

Studies using endurance athletes have suggested similar requirements to those of strength athletes, owing to the vast amount of microtrauma caused by repeated repetitions on the road or bike. Athletes participating in at least 2-3 bouts of endurance training a week benefit from levels of 1.8-2.0g/kg/bw (2), with higher levels preventing lean mass loss during periods of energy restriction. Retention in fat free mass during periods of targeted weight loss have been significant even in levels as high as 2.0-2.5g/kg/bw (2).

Protein intake during training has been a topic of much debate over its effectiveness to improve performance and recovery for endurance athletes. While carbohydrate intake during sessions is widely accepted as aiding performance and recovery, the effect of intra-exercise protein intake is less well understood. A study of elite level cyclists on a week-long training camp split the group into two; one consuming a carbohydrate-based drink and the other an isocaloric whey protein and carbohydrate blend. Despite it being typically believed that endurance athletes need an elevated intake of protein, results showed that muscle breakdown, immune function and power tests taken at the end of the week yielded no significant results between the groups (3). Comparisons between athletes consuming post-exercise isocaloric drinks of either carbohydrate-only, high-carb/low protein or high protein/low carbohydrate have also shown to promote similar levels of recovery and subsequent performance in endurance athletes (4).

These findings suggest that it's not so much the protein timing but the consistency of the intake over the day/week that results in sustained MPS rates. There is some evidence to suggest that supplementing with protein during exercise does impact skeletal muscle and HR response despite not showing any meaningful performance differences in cycling (5).

Protein dosing through the day is therefore an important consideration when it comes to optimal recovery, rather than timing around training per se. Knowing the ideal spread throughout the day will help athletes ensure optimal meal timings for recovery and performance. In one seminal study, men weighing roughly 80kg consumed 80g protein in a day, in either 10, 20 or 40g doses, with the 20g dosage individuals showing better results (6).

Fig. 68

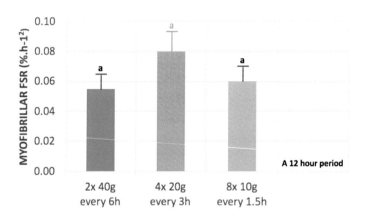

Other studies into protein dosage size and its effect on MPS rates are useful when looking at how much protein we should be having in each intake. In one, (7) subjects consumed a standardised, high-protein (0.54g/kg/body mass) breakfast. Three hours later, a bout of strength exercise was performed. Subjects then ingested either 0, 10, 20, or 40g whey protein isolate immediately (~10 min) after exercise. Control groups also followed the same protocol without the strength training. As you'd expect, MPS rates did not increase significantly with the groups on 0g of protein, and while the group on 10g of protein showed increases in MPS, these were not within rates of statistical significance.

Fig. 69

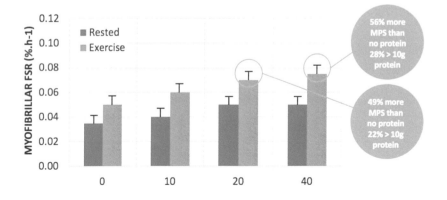

The non-active groups' MPS rates (blue bars) reached their peak at around 20g per serving, with larger doses yielding no benefit. The exercised individuals (orange bar) showed MPS rate increases of 49% and 56% for 20g and 40g groups respectively. The 40g dose saw an increase in amino acid oxidation & ureagenesis; converting of amino acids into urea, which for only a 7% increase in MPS is a very small return for twice the amount of protein. One could argue that this is a small price to pay and we have previously recommended opting for the higher figure when looking to maximise hypertrophy, but this is nonetheless food for thought and while it's still a good idea to recommend clients aim for the higher dose of roughly 40g protein, or 0.55g/kg of bodyweight per meal previously highlighted, halving this intake is not the end of the world. Additionally, it's worth noting that 20-40g is a large jump, and it would be interesting to see how much of that 7% increase occurs at 30g.

Of course, to fully optimise recovery from endurance training, recovery strategies should ensure adequate intake of carbohydrate as well as protein, to enable glycogen synthesis and muscle protein synthesis respectively. Consuming both after training is a very good idea but one should be careful not to neglect carbohydrates during the rest of the day, too, as it's not only difficult to consume huge carbohydrate doses in one sitting, but carbohydrate synthesis appears to be better achieved with multiple feedings (8).

22.9. Nutrition periodisation

"The concept of matching performance nutrition strategies to training demands to support different phases of training and competition". Lucy Wainwright, EIS Performance Nutritionist British Triathlon.

Endurance nutrition needs to be periodised just like training, as this allows your client to prioritise their goals one at a time. Depending on an athlete's given sport or discipline, their training needs will change throughout the year. For endurance athletes, in-seasonal sports may be triathlon, duathlon and cycling; while off-season training may include a greater proportion of strength work, injury prevention or rehab. Immediately after the season has ended there may be a period of very low volume training followed by a phase of more technique work and less intensity, creating a full deload. During this stage, the athlete's energy requirements may be a lot lower than during a competitive season.

Macronutrient requirements may be different too, since carbohydrate is the body's preferred fuel source for higher intensity, sustained endurance performance. If an athlete is performing lower volume and potentially lower intensity training, they might not require such a large amount of this fast-acting fuel source. Because of this, any decrease in energy intake could come primarily from a reduction in carbohydrate intake, to maintain similar protein and fat numbers. This will change athlete to athlete depending on their training styles, and their preferences. In-season, however, while preference still plays a massive role, endurance sport nutrition becomes much more grounded in physiology. To understand this, it's useful to recap the energy systems.

22.10. Energy systems and muscle fibre type

To understand more about the demands of endurance sports, we will now look at the different energy systems and how they may be relevant to these athletes. There are four different energy systems used by the body to regenerate ATP, with your reliance on each being primarily dictated by the intensity of the exercise being undertaken. They are:

- **Aerobic lipolysis:** This is fat usage in the presence of oxygen. Produces a huge amount more energy per unit of FFA than can be produced per unit of glucose. Used during very low intensity activities and can sustain many hours of activity

- **Aerobic glycolysis:** Uses carbohydrate in the form of glucose (from both glycogen and blood glucose) in the presence of oxygen. This allows for significantly more ATP to be produced from one unit of glucose, compared to anaerobic methods – as such, aerobic glycolysis is used for activity lasting significantly longer and is likely the key energy system in use over most competitive endurance events from 1-10 hours in duration

- **Anaerobic glycolysis:** This is the use of carbohydrate in the absence of oxygen. It fuels exercise lasting between 20-60 seconds or so. Performing anaerobic glycolysis results in the production of lactate and hydrogen (often referred to as Lactate Threshold (LT) when referring to training zones). It is often accompanied by a 'burning' sensation within the muscles. This energy system causes fatigue quickly

- **Phosphocreatine (PCr) system:** This system uses a molecule of creatine phosphate, a naturally occurring molecule within muscle tissue and is used for the first 1-20 seconds of maximal intensity exercise such as a 100m sprint or bunch sprint in cycling

It's important to remember that these energy systems are not mutually exclusive, and so there's some overlap between the systems as intensity gradually increases. It's not like a switch that suddenly changes where you're getting your energy from. While we might associate endurance sports with the first two energy systems, it's actually very common for athletes to utilise at least three of these systems, if not all of them. Even when we try to maintain a steady pace we may encounter a headwind or gradient that requires more effort to overcome and so although pace may not change, intensity does and so will the fuel source used. If this occurs an athlete will spend short durations working in their anaerobic zone to cope, then pay off that 'debt' by working back within their aerobic systems.

Think of a 10,000m track race in athletics. These are rarely run at the athlete's personal best speeds and lap times are often very inconsistent. This is because races like this are very tactical, with the pack running well within their aerobic capacity and athletes occasionally testing the pack by trying to surge in speed followed by a slowing down. The idea is to get your competitors working with their anaerobic glycolysis system and hope that you can recover more quickly so that when you surge again, they are unable to go with you. Other examples might be when an athlete hangs at the back for an entire race, working aerobically, before a huge anaerobic surge at the end. We've seen this pay off in Mo Farah's gold medal races in 2012 and 2016. When it's miscalculated, however, we see athletes slow up just before the finish line, get passed, and often finish way down the field.

In cycling, team time trials are events where teams of riders set off at intervals and must work together to complete the course in the fastest time possible. To do this, they ride in a very tight formation, utilising the aerodynamic advantages of drafting. The rider at the front will work for a calculated time using their anaerobic energy system until they reach their limit, at which point they peel off allowing the second rider in the line to take up the work. The first rider then drops to the back to the line and rests until it's their turn to go again. With aerodynamics allowing around a 30% saving in effort, this is quite a shift in energy systems. With all the technology available to professional athletes and teams these days, they can almost calculate exact power targets to the nearest second to work to, to get the most from every rider. In fact, in many events the team time is taken on the fourth rider to cross the line despite the team consisting of six riders. In this instance the athletes' strategy will be to get two of the riders to 'sacrifice' themselves until they are completely spent, at which point they drop off and finish a few minutes later.

In longer events such as Ironman triathlon, you might assume athletes are aiming to avoid working anaerobically given the extreme duration (around 8 hours for pro's and >10 hours for amateurs). However, because triathlon is a non-drafting sport, athletes must often put in shorter to moderate efforts to clear other athletes and create a gap. Other factors such as course conditions, like hills and weather, will often mean the athletes have to work for short durations in their anaerobic glycolysis system.

There are three different types of fibres within muscle, each with different characteristics that determine their function with different movements. The exact distribution of each fibre type will vary depending on different genetic factors, the particular muscle group in question, and to some degree training stimulus, although the degree to which this is possible is still debated (9). It does beg the question; does athletes' muscle fibre distribution change through training, or do we eventually stumble into sports that complement our muscle fibre type? Regardless, they can be classified into the following groups:

- Type I: "slow twitch": Slow oxidative fibres which are dense with mitochondria, making them ideal for aerobic glycolysis and lipolysis

- Type IIa: "fast twitch": Fast oxidative and glycolytic fibres, moderate levels of mitochondria which are able to contract faster than type I fibres. These fibres would typically be recruited during use of the aerobic and anaerobic glycolysis energy systems

- Type IIb (or type IIx, depending on the study in question) "fast twitch": Fast glycolytic fibres with low mitochondrial density that are capable of much greater force production. They are primarily used in the anaerobic glycolysis and phosphocreatine energy systems

As with energy systems, muscle fibre recruitments aren't an immediate switch from one to the other, but rather an addition of working motor units and their associated fibres. As we start with lower force production, perhaps over a longer duration, we start with type I, working our way up the ladder until we require more force production, at which point we start recruiting type IIa, and in turn type IIb(x). Because of their physical make up and associated energy systems, the more type II fibres we recruit the more we start to rely on glycolysis. The below figures illustrate the heart rate brackets at which muscle fibres are recruited – there is overlap so, for example, at 60% of maximum heart rate, type I fibres are still working hard. Indeed, at 50%MHR the primary muscle fibres working are still type I.

- **0-20% maximum heart rate:** Type I

- **20-65% maximum heart rate:** Type IIa

- **65-85% maximum heart rate:** Type IIb (x)

After 85% of maximal effort all fibre types are already recruited, and any further force production is a result of neural signals 'making the muscles work harder' rather than additional recruitment.

As you can see, when measuring intensity and work rates in endurance sports one of the most comparable across the board is Heart Rate (HR). It's the easiest and often the most practical to measure since monitors are inexpensive. It's also relatable to changes in fitness and form throughout the year (meaning running at a given pace will induce a lesser increase in HR as you get fitter) so by using HR zones and percentage we can ensure optimal training targets, as opposed to just using target speed or paces. An alternative would be VO2max. While MHR is simply a measure of how fast the heart can beat, VO2max is the maximum rate at which oxygen can be utilised in sub-maximal and maximal exercise. There is a linear relationship between HR and VO2 at intensities above 50% VO2max, and as such we often use HR to set specific training zones (10). There are factors affecting the exact relationship between MHR and VO2max and figures are debated, especially between trained and non-trained individuals, but it does give us a starting point for comparison and a guide to where to set training zones.

The following table (10) was created as a guide to compare the two measurements in runners:

Fig. 70

%VO$_2$max	% HRmax	Speed
>50%	>70%	Very slow (warm up, cool down, recovery)
60%	75%	Slow running (early measure of a long run, recovery day)
70%	82%	Steady running (off-season; maybe challenging for LIT runs)
80%	88%	Half marathon pace; just above marathon pace
90%	95%	10k speed
95%	98%	5k speed
100%	100%	3k speed
110%	100%	1500 speed

This tells us that an athlete running at 70% MHR or less will be using fat and carbohydrate primarily for fuel, with their type I and type IIa fibres doing much of the work. At this intensity the exercise is well fuelled by fatty acids and so large carbohydrate intakes will not be needed, but as intensity increases so will reliance on type II fibres, and thus reliance on carbohydrate.

In short, carbohydrate is a necessary component of prolonged exercise intensity. This is our justification for the previous recommendation of using carbohydrates primarily to fuel endurance exercise. This idea has been challenged in recent years, so we will now look to the idea of low carbohydrate performance nutrition.

22.11. Ketogenic diets and endurance performance

Low carbohydrate or ketogenic diets continue to grow in popularity. This subject will be covered in much more detail later in the academy so for now we are going to look purely at their implementation for endurance athletes and particularly sports performance.

The biggest draw to low carbohydrate/high fat (ketogenic) diets for sports performance is the idea that if we can 'tap in' to the body's fat stores, we have an almost limitless amount of energy we can use, unlike our limited carbohydrate stores. This would prevent what runners call 'bonking', 'hitting the wall' or, more accurately, running out of fuel. It sounds great in theory, but it's not simple.

At lower intensities (up to 65% MHR) the primary source of energy is FFA thanks to the aerobic lipolysis that is used within type I muscle fibres. Endurance racing can also be fuelled with blood glucose and muscle glycogen thanks to aerobic glycolysis in both type I and type IIa fibres. As intensity increases up to 75% of MHR our demand for energy cannot be totally met from fat and we start to use more glycogen. Beyond 75% MHR, anaerobic glycolysis will be used to fuel the type II fibres. As work rate continues to increase an athlete will reach their LT at which point anaerobic energy production becomes more prominent within the body.

Increasing an athlete's LT allows them to work harder while still using aerobic energy production. Training methodology is the best way to improve this, but there is evidence that Ketogenic dieting can also increase LT (11). This is very promising at first glance for ultra-endurance or multi-day events. However, most endurance sports are not performed solely via aerobic energy systems. If a ketogenic diet deprives the body of carbohydrate then recruitment of type II fibres won't be possible, at least not for very long.

While half-marathons and marathons are still very firmly in the endurance category, they are still raced at intensities higher than ketogenic diets can cater for. A half-marathon may be performed at around 85% MHR with marathons around 75% MHR. Looking at triathlon; standard distance races are partly raced at around 90-95% MHR, meaning athletes are spending a significant duration of the race working very close to their LT, something that ketogenic dieting would not allow.

Other aspects of endurance racing that ketogenic dieting may not support include hill climbs, especially mountain top finishes, chasing a breakaway or making a sprint for the finish line.

Ketogenic diets are optimised for submaximal efforts (12, 13). Even with a fat adaptation/carbohydrate restoration model, over 100mile time trial, there was no increase in ability. In fact, it led to reduced ability in multiple sprint setting. Given the restrictions necessary to become 'fat adapted', for no significant improvement in performance one might argue the point of trying to utilise ketogenic dieting anyway. Especially when you consider that higher intensity bursts and sprint efforts that relate to most endurance sports require higher carbohydrate intake.

22.12. Fasted training for endurance performance

Training fasted has been linked to increases in PGC-1 (alpha) which is involved in mitochondrial biogenesis (14). The more mitochondria we have available, the more energy production can occur within the muscle. Training in a fasted state has been shown to improve insulin sensitivity, as well as the body's ability to continue using fat as a dominant fuel source at sub-maximal intensities.

A key factor in determining which fuel source you're using is the % of your VO2max that you're working at. Typically, around 65% of VO2max is the limit to where fat is being effectively used as fuel in exercise. Above 85% of VO2max, carbohydrate oxidation limits the fatty acid transport into mitochondria, as carbohydrate becomes the preferred fuel source at higher intensities (15). HIIT training improves our ability to work at higher intensities because of improvements in carbohydrate oxidation in the mitochondria, useful in sporting situations requiring sustained efforts. However, increasing an athlete's VO2max as well as their ability to utilise fat as a fuel source at higher rates of VO2max will mean they are able to utilise both fuel sources more effectively.

If you consider the efforts required in endurance sports; holding a threshold pace, racing in a pack and taking turns at the front, climbing a hill, environmental conditions (wind) etc. all may require working at different intensities. An athlete's ability to take advantage of this will determine their success. Methods of doing this are explained in the next section.

22.13. Metabolic flexibility and insulin resistance

Metabolic flexibility is the capacity to match fuel oxidation to fuel availability. In simple terms this means, being able to switch between fuel sources depending on what is available. As noted, the body's preferred fuel source during activity will depend on the intensity (16) and so as intensities change, it's useful to be able to switch quickly. Training effect and adaptations will improve VO2max and LT, therefore increasing the output we can create for a given HR and that fasted cardio may also help utilisation of fat usage at for longer as intensity increases (17). For the endurance athlete this means that if they can utilise fat as fuel source for a larger percentage of their MHR, they will be require less carbohydrate. In turn this means less in-race fuelling which may reduce gastric issues associated with trying to take on large amounts of fuel while competing. Being able to switch between fuel sources is important for performance since most endurance events will have variations in work rate, particularly events between 2-10 hours where athletes are working just below LT for long durations.

When looking at energy systems used by athletes, it's worth noting differences between trained vs. untrained individuals, since it's likely that more highly trained individuals will be better at switching between fuel sources. More athletic individuals, training towards a specific target are likely to include high intensity training into their endurance routine such as track and speed work. This improves recruitment of type IIa muscle fibres, required for working at higher percentage of MHR. Interval/high intensity training promotes mitochondrial adaptations to oxidise carbohydrate over fatty acids to provide energy more readily (18).

A common factor influencing metabolic flexibility is insulin resistance, associated with obesity. Chronically elevated insulin levels related to continuous overeating result in tissues becoming more resistant to the effects of insulin, and therefore they do not absorb glucose properly from the bloodstream. In reaction, the body releases higher levels of insulin and the cycle continues until the beta cells of the pancreas become damaged, eventually culminating in type 2 diabetes. Working to improve metabolic flexibility through fasted training may help improve insulin sensitivity (19), though the primary concern here should still be weight loss and a generally active lifestyle.

Popular methods of improving an athlete's ability to use fats as a fuel source is the 'train low, compete high' approach, where carbohydrate intake is significantly lower during training periods and then increased in the build-up to a race. In theory the athlete will become more used to working with lower levels of carbohydrate in their bodies and then in competition when the body needs it, it will be more available. The biggest issue with this model is that, as we've already discussed; restricting carbohydrate will limit one's ability to work at LT and above, meaning that higher intensity training will be affected. Endurance athletes, even those competing in events well over 6 hours, will still work on speed and power. Training may include short sprint repeats in the pool, track sessions, intervals on the bike, hill reps etc., all of which improve their ability to perform periods of harder work during a race. If the quality of these sessions suffers through restrictive dieting, then their effectiveness for race preparation will be greatly reduced.

A better approach is to utilise fasted, or semi-fasted training. Methods for doing this include:

- Performing interval training in the evening, consuming a low carbohydrate evening meal, waking and then doing a longer, slower run in the fasted state

- Performing interval training in the morning to deplete glycogen, consuming no carbohydrate, then performing a longer, slower run in the evening before refuelling

The approach chosen will always depend on the athlete, but overall attempts to improve metabolic flexibility may help improve endurance performance. While well trained athletes already near optimal bodyweight may have sufficient ability to do this, there may be benefit in improving utilisation of aerobic lipolysis (burning fat as fuel) for beginner athletes or those who may be looking to reduce weight as well as combat some level of insulin resistance.

22.14. Race week, the taper and carbohydrate (CHO) loading

A taper phase is a reduction in training volume over a variable time to allow physiological and psychological recovery from training to ensure optimal performance. The distance and type of event being undertaken, as well as athlete experience, will determine the level of taper. Generally speaking shorter events require a shorter lead in taper because training volumes are already lower. Maintaining training intensity is essential to avoid loss in performance leading up to a race.

The type of event will also determine the taper, for example swimming is less stressful to the body than running so you could argue this requires less of a taper. Less experienced athletes may not be training at as high intensity as their more experienced counterparts so it can be argued they may require a shorter taper. The other advantage of a shorter taper is that less experienced athletes may have less honed motor patterns for sport, especially in very skill based activities such as swimming, so we may argue that continuing training, albeit at a reduced volume right up until racing, will ensure a greater performance.

All of these factors will determine how you design your athlete's taper and therefore what considerations you need to make when designing their race week nutrition protocol. Tapering is also when we look at ensuring our bodies are optimally fuelled for performance and glycogen stores are full. This is also known as carbohydrate loading.

Carbohydrate loading is a big topic in endurance performance and one about which attracts some contradicting views. The principal is simple; to ensure that muscles are recovered and sufficiently saturated with glycogen to provide an athlete with greater endurance performance. But just what is the best way to do this? Early models of carbohydrate loading were developed in the late 1960's and typically involved a 3-4 day 'depletion phase' of hard training plus a low carbohydrate diet. This depletion phase was thought to be necessary to stimulate the enzyme glycogen synthase. This was then followed immediately by a 3-4 day 'loading phase' involving rest combined with a high carbohydrate diet. The combination of the two phases was shown to boost muscle carbohydrate stores beyond their usual resting levels.

Modern adaptations of this protocol have largely done away with the depletion phase as it was shown to be difficult for athletes to sustain useful training during this time. Plus, it's not great for an athlete's psychology to be feeling that low in the build-up to a race. The Australian Institute of Sport (20) recommends carbohydrate loading take place over 1-3 days before competition but may be compromised if the taper is not sufficient. In order to consume enough carbohydrate, it is recommended that a larger proportion comes from lower fibre sources to reduce the chances of stomach upset, especially in the final 24 hours before a race.

The amount of carbohydrate that is normally stored in the body of a given individual is dependent on diet and athletic conditioning level. For an untrained individual consuming a high carbohydrate (75%) diet, glycogen stores may be up to 130g and 360g for liver and muscle respectively for a total storage of 490g. For an athlete training daily and consuming a lower carbohydrate diet (45%), glycogen levels typically approximate 55g and 280g for liver and muscle respectively yielding a total of 330g – depleted due to a lower intake and higher output. However, should this same well-conditioned athlete consume a high carbohydrate diet (75%), their total carbohydrate reserves may soar up to 880g with approx. 160g stored in the liver and 720g in the muscle. So, the conditioned athlete's muscles are more efficient at storing carbohydrates than those of their un-conditioned competitor. This is due to altered enzymatic activity and muscle insulin sensitivity.

More recently, research has demonstrated that the glycogen stripping method may not in fact be necessary at all to achieve optimal carbohydrate saturation in well-trained individuals, and that if a lower carbohydrate intake is used, this super compensation effect may not even occur. Studies have demonstrated that athletes simply consuming a high carbohydrate diet (75%) for three days prior to competition saw carbohydrate stores comparable to those individuals who performed the glycogen stripping method. This means that the modern approach to carbohydrate loading is far less complex than it once was – this will be properly explained in a later section. It's worth noting at this stage that the overall caloric intake doesn't need to be increased significantly during a taper and carbohydrate load, since an energy buffer will already be created by reduced training stress (21).

22.15. Caution with carbohydrate loading

While the advantages of having fully saturated muscles for endurance performance are clear, there are some disadvantages and risks. Firstly, glycogen storage is linked to concomitant storage of water. It is estimated that every gram of glycogen stored is associated with about 2.7g of water. Therefore, a well-conditioned athlete with total glycogen stores approaching 800g will find their body weight about 2kg heavier at the start of the race. This increased body weight will have implications on running economy and performance, at least near the beginning of the event when energy reserves will be high. A possible solution to the water retention and weight gain is for the athlete to load to a lesser degree and ingest a carbohydrate/electrolyte enriched drink during exercise to help maintain blood glucose and electrolyte balance.

Another drawback to carbohydrate loading if performed incorrectly is gastric/intestinal upset. Very large amounts of ingested carbohydrate can affect the osmolality of the intestine. In other words, carbohydrates (especially simple/processed sugars) in the intestine draw water into the gut by osmosis affecting the water balance and may cause intestinal upset and diarrhoea. Ultimately, the only way to get this right from athlete to athlete is start with these guidelines and use trial and error to work out what works and what doesn't.

22.16. Modern adaptations

Carbohydrate loading for events lasting less than 90 minutes is not considered necessary. However, you'd still want to make sure an athlete is fully recovered and fuelled enough for the event. You could adopt a "no load" by simply maintaining a regular training diet in terms of macros but taper training a little to help a full recovery.

It is suggested that it is the amount, rather than the nature of the carbohydrate consumed during a 3-day isoenergetic carbohydrate loading (calories remain the same but macro ratios favour carbohydrates) may be the most overriding factor on subsequent metabolism and endurance run performance (22). Therefore, during the taper phase an athlete may maintain their energy intake as normal, allowing the reduced training load to create a calorie surplus that should replenish muscle glycogen. From here, altering of the percentage intake of carbohydrate can be done to match the athletes' requirements. For example, if an athlete is consuming 6g of carbohydrate per kg/bw, this may increase to 10g, with a reduction in fat and protein to compensate during a carbohydrate loading protocol.

Using the AIS recommendations (20) for events lasting <90 minutes; 7-12g of carbohydrate should be consumed per kg/bw for 24 hours, and for events >90 minutes in duration athletes should increase their carbohydrate intake to 10-12 g /kg/bw weight for 36-48 hours before race start.

Tapering towards your race should be sufficient for most of your client's energy recovery and soft tissue repair. The attention should really fall towards food sourcing rather than quantity. Take away tips are:

- Protein content in food is largely the same, but perhaps a smaller % of overall diet, 1.6-1.8 g/kg/bw

- Carbohydrate intake should increase to 7-12g/kg/bw depending on race duration

- Carbohydrate type. Complex varied carbohydrate sources for the week moving into higher Glycaemic Index (GI) foods the day before and avoiding fibre in the morning to prevent gastric issues. This will vary client to client and trial and error is the only means of actually determining what will work

22.17. How much is enough?

Just because once race might be longer than another, it doesn't mean the amount of loading for that event increases linearly. You can only fill what you have, and an athletes' total storage capacity is going to be the same regardless of the race distance. The difficulty in-race fuelling comes at the point where we race in events that require more energy than we can store. The table below shows the estimated energy stores in humans (23).

22.18. Estimated energy stores in humans

Fig. 71

Energy source	Storage site	Approximate energy (kcal)
ATC/CP*	Various tissues	5
Carbohydrate	Blood glucose	80
	Liver glycogen	400
	Muscle glycogen	1500
Fat	Serum free fatty acids	7
	Serum triglycerides	75
	Muscle triglycerides	2500
	Adipose tissue	80000+
Protein	Muscle protein	30000

*ATP/CP = adenosine triphosphate/creatine phosphate.

With obvious differences depending on storage efficiency, there's a broadly accepted and quoted figure of approximately 2000kcal of usable carbohydrate within our bodies (increasing to perhaps 3500kcal after loading), and how quickly we use that is determined by our efficiency and intensity of exercise.

Our fuel tank has a limit and once it's full it's full. If you're competing in an ultra-endurance event; double marathon, Ironman, or long sportive rides then you are probably going to empty this tank no matter how you load the week before. Any event where you are likely to be transitioning from stored energy to a reliance on intra-race fuelling could arguably be fuelled for in the same way. And in terms of how you prepare for that race, the key is to make sure you experience this in training, so you have an idea of when this happens and how to best cope with it. This is when your race day nutrition strategy is key.

22.19. Race day nutrition

For this section we assume loading has been done as per the above, 10-12g/kg for the two days before racing.

Your day should start with a small, easy to digest breakfast that's aimed at topping up your glycogen stores and blood sugar ahead of your race. Pick foods that sit well with you and that you've tried and tested in training. For short races we would recommend something small and easy to digest, such as a banana, energy bar and a protein smoothie, or even a bowl of Rice Krispies around 1-4 hours beforehand, depending how much you have and how far you're racing. For longer races, how much you can eat is trial and error, but if you're going long distance then you'll have mid-race fuelling to think about also.

22.20. In-race fuelling

Mid-race fuelling is the balance between energy output and energy intake, with the limiting factors being the speed at which nutrients can be absorbed and utilised. This is affected by %MHR of activity, with higher heart rates drawing blood away from the digestive system as well as individual ability to process food in the gut.

For endurance events, The Australian Institute of Sport recommends the following guidelines for in-event fuelling (20):

Fig. 72

<45min	Not required
45-75min	Small amounts including mouth rinse
1-2.5h	30-60g/hr
2.5-3h	Up to 90g/hr using multiple transportable carbohydrates e.g. glucose:fructose mix

These guidelines provide a starting point, with the athletes' tolerance being the determining factor in how much they can consume. There are two main limiting factors to performance in endurance sport. Firstly, biomechanical efficiency and robustness, which will determine just how hard the body can work before muscle damage and joint inflammation reduce efficiency and secondly; the athlete's ability to absorb energy on the go, which comes down to in part to the rate of gastric emptying. In ultra-distance events such as the UTMB which is a 168km trail run with 9,600m of climbing over Mont Blanc, sometimes the requirement for fuel is high but the body struggles to process anything. While before the race athletes will consume the sort of carbohydrate loading diet we'd expect to see, during the event is a different matter. One example of an athlete who completed this race in just under 26h 50m, reported that by the half way stage he was pretty much only able to consume soup and flat Coca Cola at the aid stations.

The race distance will determine how much energy you consume, as will the sport. Obviously the longer the event, the more energy you need. If you think about the marathon it's around the 20 mile mark is when you hear about people 'hitting the wall', that moment when there's nothing left in the tank. Because running typically burns a little more energy per hour than cycling, and in turn cycling more than swimming, it can be tricky trying to work out just how long our energy stores will last.

So how can we calculate our energy requirements more personally? For those looking to spend a lot of money, there are many human performance laboratories around the country where you can pay to have any number of tests carried out from HR, sweat rate, sweat-salt concentration, LT, power, running/cycling economy etc. But the easiest way is to use the training and race data from training apps and wearable devices such as Garmin.

Using the current author as an example, the table below shows three competitive swims, rides and runs, their calorie expenditure per minute and the average expected expenditure per hour for each. The swim data is taken without HR information, so the watch must estimate, based on distance and time. What this gives us is a starting point to be able to predict the caloric cost of a race and when we need to start replacing calories. For single discipline athletes this will allow you to plan a fairly linear fuel replacement strategy based on race distance and expected energy expenditure.

Fig. 73

Swim				Bike				Run			
Dist.	Time	Kcal	Kcal/min	Dist.	Time	Kcal	Kcal/min	Dist.	Time	Kcal	Kcal/min
1	00.21.49	478	21.9	1	01.12.48	949	13.2	1	00.38.08	694	18.3
2	00.22.29	582	25.8	2	01.08.38	1057	15.4	2	01.10.29	1204	17.1
3	00.23.18	536	23	3	01.13.41	1070	14.5	3	00.40.18	796	19.8
		Av.	23.6			Av.	14.4			Av.	18.4
		Kcal/HR	1414			Kcal/HR	862			Kcal/HR	1104

Using the above, note that an athlete will have 2-3500kcal stored roughly depending on the amount of carbohydrate loading that has been done, we can see that the athlete will 'hit the wall' after roughly two hours. In order to maintain maximum performance therefore, consuming energy after the one hour mark will be important. The kind of carbohydrate needs to be carefully planned, however, because consuming carbohydrate isn't what is needed – absorbing it is.

22.21. Carbohydrate types and gastric emptying rates

Factors affecting the rate of gastric emptying include (but are not limited to), the caloric content of the drink, volume, osmolality, temperature, pH, metabolic state and ambient temperature. The most important variable appears to be caloric content, with higher concentrations reducing emptying rates. At sub-maximal exercise (<75% VO2max) gastric emptying occurs at much the same rate as at rest, with it being inhibited with increases in intensity (24).

Carbohydrate blends in sports drinks are nothing new but are usually touted for their dual release properties. This property reduces the spikes and drops in blood sugar, resulting in a more gradual energy release as they're taken during activity. In addition to this there are a plethora of studies (25) suggesting that multiple transportable carbohydrates enhance gastric emptying and fluid delivery, when comparing glucose:fructose solutions with glucose alone and water. These same results have been replicated using other combinations including fructose:maltodextrin, (26) and glucose:maltodextrin. These combinations can also increase in carbohydrate oxidation rates than when taking a single source carbohydrate.

Another source of fuelling slowly making a mark are Highly Branched Cyclic Dextrin (HBCD) which benefit endurance sports for the following reasons; reduction in stress hormone production following exhaustive exercise (27), higher rates of gastric emptying especially under lower osmotic pressure (28) and reduced rate of perceived exertion with HBCD compared to maltodextrin (29).

The majority of sports nutrition products aimed at in-event fuelling for endurance athletes consist of these dual carbohydrate blends. Some of them also add in extra electrolytes to replenish those lost from sweat. However, while energy demands will be similar for the same race distance completed in different climates, the demands for electrolytes may change. As a rule of thumb, it's best to try a selection of different nutrition products in isolation in training to rule out any that may disagree with the athlete's stomach. From here it's then trial and error to work out exact fuelling strategies.

22.22. Logistics in-race fuelling and examples

As athletes and coaches, once we have calculated the energy requirements for completing a given event or race, the next thing to consider is how to implement that fuelling strategy. It isn't as simple as just spreading intake evenly over the race duration as there may be other factors to consider.

Because the body will use the fuel source that it the most readily available, once we start taking on nutrition during training or an event, our bodies will make use of the increased blood glucose in favour of stored energy. As such we do not need to take on any energy until somewhere between 60-90 minutes into activity, other than perhaps water or electrolytes depending on environmental conditions.

Single sport events like a marathon may be the closest one gets to being able to fuel on a fairly strict schedule. In this instance, once you've calculated the intake required to ensure an athlete can finish the race, it's a case of spreading it at 20-30 minute intervals from the first intake.

External factors that may affect your fuelling strategy include the course, environmental conditions and the distribution of aid stations. Technically demanding or hilly courses will dictate where the most effort will be spent, which in turn may establish where an athlete would be fuelling. For example, taking on too much fuel before trying to put in a big effort may cause discomfort. Temperature will affect how much water will need to be consumed, which may determine the concentration of carbohydrate drink that should be taken. Hotter events that require more water intake may mean you have to consume a lower percentage carbohydrate drink to allow high liquid intake without over fuelling. Event organisers will place aid stations along the route, but the frequency will differ from race to race. The more aid stations there are, the less the athlete may have to carry on their own, instead being able to factor in replacing water and some energy at each station.

Multi-sport events bring with them new considerations for fuelling. In triathlon most of the fuelling is done on the bike since you are able to both carry and consume more fuel than anywhere else in the race. The smoother movement of the bike, combined with its longer duration and being able to store and carry more, makes this the easiest place to fuel. In shorter races just a carbohydrate drink and or an energy gel may be enough to get an athlete to the end of a race. For longer distance racing athletes will require energy intake on the bike and the run in order to finish. Instead of an even spread over the race duration, many athletes may choose to over fuel slightly on the bike to allow them to take on slightly less on the run, when they different movement and increased fatigue may slow gastric emptying rate. Common types of energy taken on by athletes in races include carbohydrate drinks, gels and bars. This offers a choice of liquids or solids depending on what the athlete prefers. This may be dictated by what sits well in their stomach, or what they prefer at a given time. Rotating the sources for some may take the strain off having to consume so much. It is advised that all race nutrition is thoroughly tested in training before being implemented in a race situation. It's always worth having a plan-B however; if all else fails, eat what you can when you can and just get to the end of the race.

A fairly new multi-sport that's rising in popularity over the last decade is swim-run. Unlike aquathlon which consists of a single swim and then a run with only a single transition and is usually a shorter distance sport, swim run consists of multiple swims and runs spready over longer distances. Breca Buttermere is a good example of this; a race consisting of 38km of running and 6 km of swimming, spread over 17 different legs, athletes are constantly switching between swimming and running over mixed terrain, with all your kit with you the whole time. Athletes wear specially adapted amphibious wetsuits which are worn for swimming and running as well as keeping their shoes on the whole time. One off the biggest logistical issues here is that you have 3-4 aid stations plus whatever you are willing to carry with you. The more you carry, the more choice you may have but the extra weight and bulk you'll be running and swimming with. Challenging terrain and sporadic aid stations mean that you can't always take on nutrition or hydration at small evenly distributed intervals, so a race plan needs to be developed to cope with this.

When planning your athlete's race nutrition, work with them in training to test out different protocols and look into their races to plan strategies that can be tried out in training.

22.23. Race day supplementation

The two most commonly used and current race day supplements are probably caffeine and beetroot juice. While caffeine supplementation is nothing new there's still some debate about how best to implement it. While most studies will concur that supplementing with caffeine improves sports performance by decreasing rate of perceived exertion, improved fat metabolism and lower respiratory exchange ratio (30), there is some debate as to dosage and the effectiveness of withdrawal or abstinence prior to use. Some suggest that the performance benefits of caffeine are increased in habitual caffeine users and so they should go without caffeine for 5-7 days.

A dose of 3 mg/kg elicits improved performance regardless of whether a four day withdrawal is undertaken or not (31). Other studies also support this suggesting that it's the dosage rather than the withdrawal that's the key factor. However, it might be advisable to abstain from caffeine prior to use on race day as it Improves sleep quality in the build-up to a race.

Beetroot is one of the densest sources of nitrate, which have been shown to have benefits for endurance sport (32, 33). Nitrate augments exercise performance via an enhanced function of type II muscle fibres, a reduced ATP cost of muscle force production, an increased efficiency of mitochondrial respiration and an increased blood flow to the muscle. There are few side effects, but there may be a potential for gastric upset for susceptible athletes and should therefore be tested thoroughly in training before being implemented as part of a race strategy (34).

22.24. Relative Energy Deficiency in Sport (RED-S)

RED-S is a more modern term derived from what was formally known as The Female Athlete Triad. The female athlete triad is a syndrome that is associated with three interrelated conditions, which if allowed to become severe enough will put female athletes' health and performance at risk. The triad consists of; operating in an energy deficit (with or without disordered eating) which is the primary cause of the condition, and the two primary results, irregular menstrual function and a loss in bone mineral density (35).

The RED-S model was developed to be more comprehensive in addressing parallel occurrences of risks to health in male and female athletes. The physiological systems affected include but are not limited to; metabolism, menstrual function, bone health, immunity, protein synthesis, and cardiovascular health caused by relative energy deficiency. This energy deficiency is relative to the balance between dietary energy intake and expenditure required for health, growth activity involved in daily living as well as athletic energy expenditure. Psychological consequences may precede RED-S or be a result of it.

Low energy availability, either through low intake or increase expenditure, causes adjustments to the body's systems to reduce energy expenditure which may lead to a disruption of an array of hormonal and metabolic functions.

Some of the causes of RED-S relate to energy imbalances which may occur through disordered eating or simply as a result of failing to replace energy expended through training. It's for this reason that it can be difficult to spot initially. Disordered eating may start with appropriate eating behaviours including healthy dieting and progress into abnormal eating behaviours associated with body image and variable athletic performance.

Being able to identify RED-S at an early stage is critical for minimising long-term affects to athlete health. Many of the symptoms may need to be diagnosed clinically, which might not always be easily available to amateur athletes and coaches. However, since low energy availability plays arguably the most significant role in RED-S, any diagnosis should focus on identifying any energy imbalance and the reasons for them.

22.25. Health consequences of RED-S

Given the vastness of this topic and the degree to which it may affect an athlete's health, we recommend familiarising yourself with the information provided by the IOC as well as the links in their original article, found here: http://bjsm.bmj.com/content/48/7/491.

Briefly, RED-S typically occurs in athletes with a reduced energy availability. As you know, TDEE is made up of BMR, NEAT, TEF and EAT, and each of these components cannot properly occur without adequate energy being available for it. Athletes experience RED-S because, simply, a low energy intake is combined with a large amount of EAT. Of course, NEAT and TEF will be reduced due to this low intake as the body tries to compensate for the deficiency but eventually a number of the functions associated with BMR will be impaired, too, resulting in all of the above physiological and psychological issues.

Energy availability is defined as energy intake, minus energy expenditure through exercise, expressed as calorie per kilogram of fat free mass. To illustrate here's an example:

- Athlete is 70kg and 15% bodyfat, meaning they have roughly 60kg of fat free mass
- Athlete consumes 2700kcal per day
- Athlete expends on average 600kcal per day when calculated across the week
- Athlete has 2100kcal available for BMR, TEF and NEAT
- 2100/60 is 35, meaning the athlete has an energy availability of 35kcal/kg/FFM

The IOC state that energy balance is achieved with an energy availability of roughly 45kcal/kg/FFM and note that serious health consequences occur at a chronic intake of less than 30kcal/kg/FFM. While this level of intake may be necessary for individuals seeking to lose fat over the short-term, this is a level that represents a compromise to health for athletes seeking to perform and so should be considered a rough cut-off point for energy intake in endurance athletes.

22.26. Summary

The nutritional requirements of endurance athletes are relatively straightforward but that does not mean that they can be taken lightly. Ensuring these athletes achieve calorie sufficiency should be the first port of call, with that being achieved through adequate carbohydrate intake first and foremost due to the nature of the sport itself. That does not, however, mean that protein and fat can be ignored.

Calorie needs will vary day to day, but this does not necessarily indicate that intake does. Instead it is a reasonable and often desirable option to average energy needs out over a longer period and have a client eat roughly the same amount each day. This makes energy sufficiency easier to achieve and will thus improve adherence in many cases. Achieving energy sufficiency will not only improve performance and recovery but is the primary strategy for avoiding RED-S and the associated health complications.

Beyond that, carbohydrate loading and in-race fuelling become important for events lasting over 60 minutes, and so the consumption of multiple-transport carbohydrates should be encouraged at a dosage appropriate to the athlete, the sport and the event in question.

22.27. References

1. Philips & Van Loon (2011) Dietary Protein for Athletes: from requirements to optimum adaptation, Journal of Sport Science; 29 Suppl 1:S29-38 [Internet] Available from: https://www.ncbi.nlm.nih.gov/pubmed/22150425.

2. Pasiakos et al. (2013) Effects of high-protein diets on fat-free mass and muscle protein synthesis following weight loss: a randomized controlled trial. The FASEB Journal, 27(9), 3837-3847 [Internet] Available from: https://www.ncbi.nlm.nih.gov/pubmed/23739654.

3. Hansen M. et al. (2016) Protein intake during training sessions has no effect on performance and recovery during a strenuous training camp for elite cyclists, Journal of the International Society of Sports Nutrition, Mar 5;13:9 [Internet] Available from: https://www.ncbi.nlm.nih.gov/pubmed/26949378.

4. Goh Q (2012) Recovery from cycling exercise: effects of carbohydrate and protein beverages, Nutrients, Jul;4(7):568-84, [Internet] Available from: https://www.ncbi.nlm.nih.gov/pubmed/22852050.

5. D'Lugos et al. (2016) Supplemental Protein during Heavy Cycling Training and Recovery Impacts Skeletal Muscle and Heart Rate Responses but Not Performance, Nutrients. Sep 7;8(9). [Internet] Available from: https://www.ncbi.nlm.nih.gov/pubmed/27618091.

6. Areta et al. (2013) Timing and distribution of protein ingestion during prolonged recovery from resistance exercise alters myofibrillar protein synthesis, The Journal of Physiology, May 1;591(Pt 9): p 2319-31 [Internet] Available from: https://www.ncbi.nlm.nih.gov/pubmed/23459753.

7. Witard et al. (2014) Myofibrillar muscle protein synthesis rates subsequent to a meal in response to increasing doses of whey protein at rest and after resistance exercise, The American Journal of Clinical Nutrition ;99 (1): p 86-95 [Internet] Available from: https://academic.oup.com/ajcn/article/99/1/86/4577382.

8. Moore, D. R. (2015). Nutrition to support recovery from endurance exercise: optimal carbohydrate and protein replacement. Current Sports Medicine Reports, 14(4), 294-300. [Internet] Available from: https://www.ncbi.nlm.nih.gov/pubmed/26166054.

9. Wilson et al. (2012) The effects of endurance, strength, and power training on muscle fibre type shifting, Journal of Strength Conditioning Research, vol. 26 (6), pages 1724-9. [Internet] Available from: https://www.ncbi.nlm.nih.gov/pubmed/21912291.

10. Swain D. Et al (1994) Target heart rates for the development of cardiorespiratory fitness, Medicine and Science in Sports and Exercise, Jan;26(1):112-6. [Internet] Available from: https://www.ncbi.nlm.nih.gov/pubmed/8133731.

11. Zajac et al. (2014) The Effects of a Ketogenic Diet on Exercise Metabolism and Physical Performance in Off-Road Cyclists, Nutrients, 6(7): p 2493–2508. [Internet] Available from: https://www.ncbi.nlm.nih.gov/pubmed/24979615.

12. Kiens (2001) Diet and training in the week before competition, Canadian Journal of Applied Physiology, 2001;26 Suppl:S56-63. [Internet] Available from: https://www. ncbi.nlm.nih.gov/pubmed/11897883.

13. Burke & Kiens (2006) "Fat adaptation" for athletic performance: the nail in the coffin? Journal of Applied Physiology, vol. 100 (1), p 7-8, [Internet] Available from: https://www.physiology.org/doi/full/10.1152/japplphysiol.01238.2005.

14. Psilanderet al. (2013) Exercise with low glycogen increases PGC-1α gene expression in human skeletal muscle. European Journal of Applied Physiology, 2013 Apr;113(4):951-63 [Internet] Available from: https://www.ncbi.nlm.nih.gov/pubmed/23053125.

15. Fernandez-Marcos & Auwerx (2011) Regulation of PGC-1α, a nodal regulator of mitochondrial biogenesis, American Journal of Clinical Nutrition, Vol. 93 (4) [Internet] Available from: https://www.ncbi.nlm.nih.gov/pubmed/21289221.

16. Galgani, Moro & Ravussin (2008) Metabolic flexibility and insulin resistance, American Journal of Physiology Endocrinology and Metabolism, 2008 Nov; vol. 295 issue 5: E1009–E1017 [Internet] Available from: https://www.ncbi.nlm.nih.gov/pubmed/ 18765680.

17. Gormley et al. (2008) Physical Fitness and Performance Effect of Intensity of Aerobic Training on VO2max, Medicine & Science in Sport & Exercise, Vol. 40, No. 7, pp. 1336-1343 [Internet] Available from: https://pdfs.semanticscholar.org/8791/89cedc5ea45 c6213d84771f2ba400bd774be.pdf

18. Daussin et al. (2008) Training at high exercise intensity promotes qualitative adaptations of mitochondrial function in human skeletal muscle, Journal of Applied Physiology, Vol. 104 no. 5, 1436-144 [Internet] Available from: https://www.ncbi. nlm.nih.gov/pubmed/18292295.

19. Van Proeyen et al. (2010) Training in the fasted state improves glucose tolerance during fat-rich diet, Journal of Physiology, Nov 1; 588: p 4289–4302 [Internet] Available from: https://www.ncbi.nlm.nih.gov/pubmed/20837645.

20. AIS Sports Nutrition (2014) Carbohydrate – The Facts [Internet] Available from: https://www.ausport.gov.au/ais/sports_nutrition/fact_sheets/carbohydrate_how_m uch

21. David Peterson, The Science of Carbohydrate Loaded, Online Article [Internet] Available from: http://www.marathontraining.com/articles/art_39th.htm.

22. Chen et al. (2008) Effect of carbohydrate loading patterns on running performance, International Journal of Sports Medicine, Jul;29(7):598-606. [Internet] Available from: https://www.ncbi.nlm.nih.gov/pubmed/18004688.

23. Suzanna Girard Eberle (2014) Endurance Sports Nutrition 3rd-Edition, Human Kinetics, Available from: http://www.humankinetics.com/products/all-products/Endurance-Sports-Nutrition-3rd-Edition.

24. Murray (1987) The effects of consuming carbohydrate-electrolyte beverages on gastric emptying and fluid absorption during and following exercise, Sports Medicine, Sep-Oct;4(5):322-51 [Internet] Available from: https://www.ncbi.nlm.nih.gov/pubmed/3313617.

25. Jeukendrup & Moseley (2010) Multiple transportable carbohydrates enhance gastric emptying and fluid delivery. Scandinavian Journal of Medicine and Science in Sports. 2010 Feb;20(1):112-21 [Internet] Available from: https://www.ncbi.nlm.nih.gov/pubmed/19000102.

26. O'Brien & Rowlands (2011) Fructose-maltodextrin ratio in a carbohydrate-electrolyte solution differentially affects exogenous carbohydrate oxidation rate, gut comfort, and performance, American Journal Physiology, Gastrointestinal & Liver Physiology, Jan;300(1):G181-9 [Internet] Available from: https://www.ncbi.nlm.nih.gov/pubmed/21071509.

27. Suzuki et al. (2014) Effect of a sports drink based on highly-branched cyclic dextrin on cytokine responses to exhaustive endurance exercise, Journal of Sports Medicine and Physical Fitness, Oct;54(5):622-30.

28. Takii et al. (2005) Fluids Containing a Highly Branched Cyclic Dextrin Influence the Gastric Emptying Rate, International Journal of Sports Medicine 26(4):314-9 [Internet] Available from: https://www.researchgate.net/publication/7840225_Fluids_Containing_a_Highly_Branched_Cyclic_Dextrin_Influence_the_Gastric_Emptying_Rate.

29. Furuyashiki et al. (2014) Effects of ingesting highly branched cyclic dextrin during endurance exercise on rating of perceived exertion and blood components associated with energy metabolism, Bioscience, Biotechnology and Biochemistry, vol 78 (12), Pages 2117-2119 [Internet] Available from: https://www.tandfonline.com/doi/abs/10.1080/09168451.2014.943654.

30. McNaughton (2008) The effects of caffeine ingestion on time trial cycling performance, International Journal of Sports Physiology and Performance, Vol. 3 (2), p 157-63 [Internet] Available from: https://www.ncbi.nlm.nih.gov/pubmed/19208924.

31. Irwin et al. (2011) Caffeine withdrawal and high-intensity endurance cycling performance. Journal of Sports Science, vol 29(5):509-15. [Internet] Available from: https://www.ncbi.nlm.nih.gov/pubmed/21279864.

32. Hoon et al. (2013) The effect of nitrate supplementation on exercise performance in healthy individuals: a systematic review and meta-analysis, International Journal of Sport Nutrition & Exercise Metabolism, 2013 Oct;23(5):522-32. [Internet] Available from: https://www.ncbi.nlm.nih.gov/pubmed/23580439.

33. Hoon et al. (2014) The effect of variable doses of inorganic nitrate-rich beetroot juice on simulated 2,000-m rowing performance in trained athletes, International Journal

of Sports Physiology & Performance, Jul;9(4):615-20. [Internet] Available from: https://www.ncbi.nlm.nih.gov/pubmed/24085341.

34. Maughan et al. (2018) IOC Medical and Scientific Commission reviews its position on the use of dietary supplements by elite athletes, British Journal of Sports Medicine 2018; 52 418-419 [Internet] Available from: http://bjsm.bmj.com/content/52/7/439.

35. Mountjoy et al. (2014) The IOC consensus statement: beyond the Female Athlete Triad–Relative Energy Deficiency in Sport (RED-S) British Journal of Sports Medicine, Vol 48, issue 7, Pages:491-497 [Internet] Available from: http://bjsm.bmj.com/content/48/7/491.

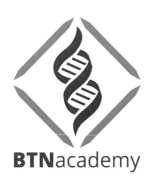

MODULE 23

ASSISTED ATHLETES

23.   MODULE 23: ASSISTED ATHLETES

23.1.   Module aims

- To provide statistics on the prevalence of steroid use in gym culture and athletics

- To give a rundown of the most commonly used steroidal drugs in gym culture, how they are used and what they do

- To provide information around other Performance Enhancing drugs (PEDs) such as clenbuterol, and DNP

- To provide basic guidance for ensuring the safety of users

- To give pros and cons of steroid use

23.2.   Key principles from module 22

In the last module we covered endurance athletes, their needs, and the strategies you can utilise to help them maximise performance. We covered:

- The main goal of endurance sport nutrition is to maintain weight while adequately fuelling for performance and recovery. This amounts to a balancing act, typically involving more precise calorie tracking than other sports and dietary goals. Weight should be monitored closely, as should subjective wellbeing

- The primary fuel for endurance athletes is carbohydrate, and carbohydrate intake thus needs to be emphasised

- Protein and fat intake are still important, however

- Carbohydrate loading is a useful strategy, with the degree of loading depending on habitual intake and the sport/event in question

- In-race nutrition should amount to simple carbohydrate in appropriate dosing, ideally from multiple different sugars (i.e. glucose and fructose)

23.3.   Introduction to assisted athletes

In this module we will turn to one of the more controversial topics pertaining to fitness: Image and Performance Enhancing Drugs (IPEDS). The purpose of this module is not to make you a drug expert, to advocate for or against the use of these compounds, nor to qualify you to start writing drug plans for clients. Of course, it also goes without saying but we will still state it clearly: we do not advise that you recommend your clients start using performance enhancing drugs, nor do we advise you do so yourself.

This module is instead here to help you understand this often mysterious side of fitness because it is unlikely that you will go through your entire career without the topic ever coming up. As you will see, drug use in gyms is increasing and their use is becoming more and more culturally normalised. This means that many clients and indeed many coaches will be tempted to experiment with them. Therefore, this module is here to give you an overview and an insight in to what these drugs do, how they work and how people use them. This will enable you to have an informed discussion if clients ever ask you your thoughts and will also simply remove a point of confusion. Reliable information is often difficult to impossible to get.

You will notice that this module is not as heavily referenced as many others and that is due to a relative lack of available research. Anabolic steroids are in essence medicines. They have specific medical uses and are sometimes prescribed to patients for a variety of reasons, and in that area, they are well researched. Steroid usage outside of this intended purpose is therefore, by definition, abuse and thanks to that, as well as a great deal of social stigma, steroid usage research in relation to resistance training is sparse. Instead this information has been largely garnered through trial and error by users in combination with evidence-based knowledge of the endocrine system, as well as some basic information about the drugs themselves. Additionally, the information below has, in places, come directly from personal conversations between the current author and the key health professionals with whom he works as the UK's leading authority on steroid harm prevention.

23.4.   What are steroids?

Anabolic androgenic steroids are synthetic compounds based on either testosterone, nandrolone or dihydrotestosterone. There are several other types of steroids including cholesterol and various medications (for example many people are given steroid creams or steroid injections to help overcome illnesses). However we are only concerned with anabolic steroids or anabolic androgenic steroids to give them their correct title in this module. These are organic compounds (meaning carbon-based), being made up of four carbon rings arranged in a specific molecular configuration. Below you see testosterone, as an example.

Fig. 74

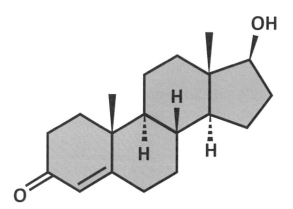

It is this specific conformation that makes the compound in question a steroid, though there are some subtle variations between different forms which allow us to differentiate between them. The word 'anabolic' refers to the drugs' muscle building properties, with anabolism being the term given to the process of biologically combining small parts into a larger whole – for example combining amino acids during protein synthesis to create muscle proteins. When testosterone, binds to a receptor on a muscle cell, that cell responds by increasing the rate at which muscle protein synthesis is performed and this is the basic way that the expected effects are caused.

'Androgenic' instead refers to many of the side effects associated with steroids. Within the human body are various sites with androgen receptors – hormone receptors to which certain things can bind (including the hormone analogues contained within the drugs in question). Once a hormone binds to one of these a given effect will be exerted, resulting in such 'male' characteristics as a deepening of the voice, increased sexual appetite, facial hair growth and accelerated balding in those prone to this. In essence because testosterone is the primary male hormone, the result of increasing it artificially is a rise in many typical male characteristics, with muscle mass being one of them.

All steroids have an anabolic to androgenic ratio, which describes the relative amount of each kind of effect that will be seen for the average person. For example, testosterone is 100/100 so is quite balanced between its muscle building properties and its side effects, whereas deca durabolin (a nandrolone steroid) is 125/37 so its effectiveness at building muscle tissue is far greater than its potential for androgenic side effects. With that being said it must be noted that these are not the only side effects that are seen! Drugs can also be considered as being aromatising or not, with this term referring to the potential for the testosterone within it to be converted into estrogen via the aromatase enzyme. High doses of aromatising compounds lead to an increase in some side effects to be listed later, and so those taking high doses of these will often require additional drugs to combat the effect. Simply, it's not the case that drugs with a high anabolic:androgenic ratio are free of side effects.

Artificially increased testosterone has many effects as you have seen, but the main ones in relation to muscle growth are, an increase in protein synthesis at the cell, the retention of nitrogen (increases protein absorption), an increase in Red Blood Cells (RBC) and a tendency to retain water. This results in the user recovering from resistance training at an accelerated rate, increasing their strength and enabling them to perform and gain muscle mass faster and beyond the natural genetic limits.

Steroids are available in injectable (both water and oil based), oral and topical cream form (cream is rarely used as a performance enhancing drug but is often prescribed for hormone replacement). In their raw state they appear as a crystallised powder which is then dissolved in a solvent and carrier oil to produce an injectable, or if orally viable the raw product is pressed into a tablet form alongside fillers. To make a steroid orally viable it must undergo a molecular conformational change, with either a methyl (one carbon and three hydrogens) or ethyl group (a combination of two carbons and five hydrogens) added to the seventeenth carbon. This prevents the compound being destroyed in first pass digestion by the liver but has important repercussions as you will see later.

These are medical supplies and therefore many drugs are produced with strict regulations (then sold on the black market) meaning that a given product is what it says on the box and at the correct dosage, but at the same time illegal bootleg manufacturers (known as underground laboratories or labs) produce copies which make up the majority of the market. These are produced without regulations or oversight, meaning they are often either under dosed, or a different product entirely to what is expected (often a cheaper yet similar compound). In recent years 'home brewing' from raw materials has become more common thanks to unreliable underground laboratory product quality.

The rise in home brewing lies at least partly in the fact that the basic production process is quite simple. You require four ingredients:

- **Raw powder:** Usually purchased from China. Underground laboratories have no facility to test what they purchase so they have no idea what they are being supplied with, nor can they test the quality/concentration of it meaning that they need to trust what the supplier tells them. In the vast majority of cases the product will be as stated but this uncertainty at the very first step should be a red flag by itself

- **Carrier oil:** Commonly, any organic oil that is liquid at room temperature. Ethyl olelate is generally considered to be the 'gold standard' but this is hard to come by, so organic grapeseed oil is typically used

- **Benzyl benzoate:** A solvent that allows the raw powder to dissolve in the carrier oil

- **Benzyl alcohol:** Sterilising agent used post-production to make sure the multi-shot vial does not get contaminated

All the brewer must do is dissolve the raw powder into the benzyl benzoate in order to allow it to mix in the carrier oil, then add the carrier until reaching the desired concentration. The amount of powder added typically ranges from 100-400mg per ml, with 250mg being the most common and anything over 500mg causing 'crashing', which means the raw powder recrystallizes and the product becomes unusable.

Once the mixture is created it is passed through a 0.22micron medical filter to sterilise it. The product is then bottled, labelled, and distributed. Vials in underground laboratories are typically multiple-use vials meaning that for example 10ml of product will be added. The user can then draw out their desired dose at a time and store again for subsequent administrations. This is as opposed to pharmaceutical manufacturers (or some more established underground laboratories) that package products in 1ml ampoules for single use. Ampoules are preferred because the glass must be broken prior to extraction, meaning that contamination risk is dramatically reduced. They are, however, far harder to make.

Fig. 75

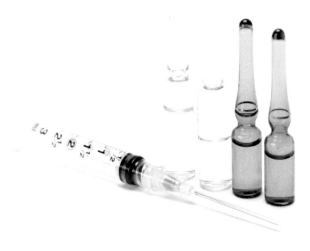

The Welsh Emerging Drugs and Identification of Novel Substances Project (3) (WEDINOS) found that 33% of the drugs they tested were not as they were labelled (unfortunately they only tested for compound presence rather than strength). Chem Clarity (a private testing service that has now ceased trading) stated that they estimated over 80% of all steroids sold via underground laboratories are incorrectly dosed.

Many users will attempt to purchase pharmaceutical products from an overseas pharmacy in countries such as Turkey or Egypt, as over-the-counter sales are legal. However many of these products are counterfeit and though may contain active ingredients they are not produced by a licenced and regulated pharmaceutical company.

23.5. The business of steroids

The production of steroids in the UK is big business. In fact, UK Anti-Doping (UKAD) regards the UK as the biggest manufacturer of illicit steroids in the world (outside of the raw powder manufacture in China). Over 496 addresses are tagged by customs at the time of writing due to the production of steroids, and recent seizures have turned up drug manufacturing facilities with in excess of 4 million pounds worth of drugs. There are roughly 200 commercial underground laboratories operating within the UK with even more people home brewing. The big incentive is money.

The manufacturing costs of drugs is exceptionally low. At the time of writing the average costs will be in the range of:

Injectables

- Testosterone: £3-7 per 10ml
- Trenbolone: £7-12 per 10ml
- Nandrolone: £3-7 per 10ml
- Masteron: £3-7 per 10ml

Orals

- Dianabol: £1-1.50 per 100
- Winstrol: £3-4 per 100
- Anavar: £7-10 per 60
- Oxymethalone: £5-7 per 60

When you compare these to the prices that are typically charged, you can see how a major profit can be made from these illegal activities (especially when you consider these individuals aren't paying tax!).

Typical trade prices for a 100 unit purchase made by a supplier:

- Testosterone: £13-17per 10ml
- Trenbolone: £17-22 per 10ml

- Nandrolone: £13-15 per 10ml

- Masteron: £13-15 per 10ml

- Dianabol: £10-12 per 100

- Winstrol: £15-20 per 100

- Anavar: £18-23 per 60

- Oxymethalone: £13-15 per 60

Typical retail price for the end user buying one vial:

- Testosterone: £30-45 per 10ml

- Trenbolone: £35-50 per 10ml

- Nandrolone: £30 -35 per 10ml

- Masteron: £25-35 per 10ml

- Dianabol: £15-25 per 100

- Winstrol: £35-50 per 100

- Anavar: £40-65 per 60

- Oxymethalone: £25-35 per 60

But who is purchasing them?

23.6.   IPED users

Clinically steroids are used for a variety of conditions including anaemia and muscle wastage disorders but by far the most common usage presently is Testosterone Replacement Therapy (TRT). Ironically a growing number of people are now genuinely requiring this thanks to the repercussions of recreational steroid abuse.

Non-clinical use is generally to increase muscle mass or athletic performance, with the former being the most popular reason outside of professional athletics. Current estimates put non-clinical steroid users in the UK at 2,000,000 users, with the vast majority of these users doing so for cosmetic rather than performance based reasons. This is primarily men seeking a greater amount of muscle mass and reduced fat mass, but the rise of Crossfit and powerlifting as well as the normalisation of steroid use in physique and even bikini competitions means that women are rapidly increasing their prevalence of use, too. On top of this there are a growing number of older men self-medicating TRT to try and combat the aging process. We can loosely group users into a number of different categories, because despite what you man initially think, steroids are not only used by bodybuilders.

23.6.1.   Competitive bodybuilders/strength sports

This has always been the most populous demographic of IPED users. Powerlifting is becoming increasingly popular, especially amongst the previously disinterested female population, and drug usage by both genders has increased to suit. Recently strongman has grown in popularity, too, and while this group have access to the same information as everybody else it is the current author's experience that this group is the least informed. The purpose of usage here primarily revolves around the ability of IPEDs to increase maximal strength through muscle hypertrophy and improved motor neuron firing, though hypertrophy, increased training recovery (meaning users can train heavier and more often without burning out) and of course aesthetics are also a factor. Additionally some drugs such as human growth hormone can improve injury recovery in certain tissues.

Bodybuilding, of course, has always been synonymous with drug use, but overall use has grown tremendously thanks to the popularity of the fitness categories. Bikini and men's physiques classes were initiated to provide a commercially viable look (something that is more achievable and more physically attractive to the mainstream than heavyweight bodybuilding) and these classes have boomed. They now provide the greatest number of competitors at shows, with the number of competitors in these classes being double that in bodybuilding.

Though the inception of these classes was to provide a natural, commercially viable looking physique, the truth is that drug use within these classes is rampant and the classes have driven female usage to its highest levels to date.

23.6.2.   Aspiring competitors

While it may seem redundant to list this group here, it is not. This is for the simple fact that many want to compete and train in order to do so (either in bodybuilding or strength sports) but never actually make the transition to competition. Drug use here is just as common, relatively speaking, but because this group far outnumbers actual competitors it is likely that they are responsible for more drug use overall.

23.6.3.   Image users

This group is by far the highest risk group, both for initiation of use and for continuation despite side effects. These are cosmetic users (those who have no interest in competing) that quite often have a very relaxed approach to drug use, and often have a cross poly drug use, which is use of, for example, anabolic steroids, fat burners, party drugs and alcohol simultaneously.

Image users are generally interested in results and not the process of attaining results, meaning their diet and training is often poor and so they have a heavy reliance on drugs, with drug use increasing as results plateau, rather than a change in programming or increase in effort. Usage is higher prior to holidays and specific events and their general lifestyles are sociable. Users choose compounds that will enhance their aesthetic appeal meaning that both anabolic and fat burner use is prized. Risk management is at best an afterthought.

Resultantly, their interaction with supportive organisations is minimal and information generally comes from peers with no real understanding of risks or potential problems arising from use. There is very little information available regarding the numbers within this user group as they make little contact with any sort of service. In fact, their interactions, even amongst forums and social media groups, are minimal. What little evidence is available about this group (word of mouth and second-hand statement) would suggest that it is very large with a very transient user base.

23.6.4.   Sports athletes

This group contains both professional and amateur sports people and has been steadily increasing over time. Usage is based around performance enhancement with many believing usage is necessary in order to perform in their chosen sport. Again, this is peer driven to a large extent but there is significant evidence that many coaches encourage usage, with a few countries even being implicated in state-sponsorship of athlete doping ahead of the Olympics. It is extremely unlikely that the countries that have already been named are the only ones doing this or similar and it would not be surprising if more stories came out in the future.

The specific drugs and desired effects will vary by sport, but the overall aim is to improve recovery from training as well as boosting performance. The drugs chosen will range from anabolic steroids to EPO which increases red blood cell count for oxygen delivery during endurance racing, and beta blockers which calm you down during shooting.

23.6.5.   Therapeutic users

This is a relatively new user group but there are increasing numbers of mature individuals turning to self-administered TRT in an attempt to counter the ageing process. There has also been an increase in growth hormone use as an anti-ageing serum within this group. Many users are 50+ and financially stable. Knowledge is poor but drug use is minimal so poses small risk and may in fact offer some genuine benefits provided users do not significantly exceed replacement dose.

Some shift workers and students will also use stimulants in an effort to stay awake and alert for longer. This has historically been relatively poorly understood, but recent Netflix documentaries that highlight ADHD medication abuse have helped bring this further into the public consciousness.

23.6.6.   Fat loss group

This user group crosses several other groups but is of increasing concern because there are significant numbers of IPED users that only use fat burners; many of whom do not realise they have bought an illicit product as its been purchased via Facebook or eBay. This user group is potentially in the millions with the number of non-exercisers that are trying to lose weight and so turning to diet pills being more significant than most would hope.

This is a group that are often overlooked (probably because they aren't using hormones) but stimulants like ephedrine and stronger fat burners like clenbuterol and DNP (both explained later) are extremely common, the latter having already caused deaths in users.

23.6.7.   Armed and emergency services

The armed services have implemented a 'with suspicion testing' service via Compulsory Drug Testing (CDT) for some years, however this form of testing is somewhat cost prohibitive and so is not done as often as it perhaps should be. The emergency services also do not test as a standard procedure and usage amongst firefighters and police offers is not uncommon.

When the typical IPED user profile is examined, user traits include those of risk taking and an interest in physical performance. This makes it somewhat self-evident that both emergency and armed services would attract people who are at high risk with regards to the potential of becoming an IPED user. Additionally, these careers combine high pressure with close-knit teams meaning that work colleagues become close friends in many instances. As drug use typically is introduced via trusted peers this allows for use to increase exponentially over time.

23.7. How steroids are used

Steroids are not typically used like supplements. While performance-based supplements such as creatine and beta alanine are used year-round, most steroid users do not use continuously and in fact doing so greatly increases the user's risk of harm. While frequency and duration of use will vary there are three typical schedules adopted:

23.7.1. Periodic cycle

This is the most common strategy. Steroids are taken for a pre-determined period of time usually in a predetermined dose with a planned recovery time-off period. Duration can range extensively, however cycles are commonly 4-16 weeks with the majority falling between 8-12 weeks. Time off is often considered to be ideally equal to time on, though some users will use far less frequently (perhaps each year in the run up to a holiday) and some will use more frequently due to fears of losing strength and size between cycles. Often this morphs into the next form of use.

23.7.2. Blast/cruise

While periodic cyclers will take a certain dose for a given amount of time and then come off, those who blast/cruise simply vary their dosage. A baseline steroid usage level is maintained, commonly around 250mg of a longer-ester drug (explained later) will be taken each week. However this can vary greatly with heavy users 'maintaining' on much more than this. The user will then dramatically increase their dose periodically. For example, a dose of 250mg of testosterone per week may be maintained year round (the cruise) with 'blast' periods of 6-12 weeks at 1500mg being included every few months.

23.8. Hormone Replacement Therapy (HRT)

This is a self-administered and self-diagnosed low dose testosterone treatment aimed at mimicking the TRT dose that would have been prescribed, had the user gone to the doctor and been tested for a genuinely low baseline testosterone level. Dosages are kept at a comparatively low 250mg per 10-14 days and maintained indefinitely (for life). HRT is generally used by older men who feel that their virility may be failing them thanks to natural declining testosterone levels.

In general, most steroid cycles are planned ahead of time and even with blast/cruises both the base line and upcoming 'blast' will be pre-determined by the user. There are a number of ways to determine the ideal dose for the individual, but it primarily comes down to trial and error, with many users starting with a 'beginner' dose at their first use and increasing dosages over time (either due to necessity because progress is no longer being made or temptation). The frequency with which a drug is administered depends on the half-life which will be fully explained later. Briefly for now, know that oral steroids as well as some injectables have an extremely short half-life and so taking daily or even multiple times per day is common; contrasted to some other injectables which can be used every week or even further apart in some cases.

The purpose of cycling rather than simply staying on all of the time is to mediate the downregulation of natural hormone levels. As steroids enter the body it senses the rise in testosterone levels and natural testosterone production ceases, (this generally takes 3-4 weeks) as testosterone levels increase oestrogen levels also rise.

High oestrogen levels can cause water retention, puberty type mood swings, gynecomastia (the development of breasts in males) and increased emotional sensitivity. To combat this, an oestrogen control drug is used, with the most common being tamoxifen citrate (Nolvadex). This blocks the oestrogen receptors from accepting the oestrogen hormone so though oestrogen is present it has little or no effect. These drugs are not often used in women because the additional oestrogen does not cause so many problems for them and in fact blocking these receptors causes issues. In fact, excessive estrogen management seems to cause significant problems for both genders, with numerous health complications (including an exacerbation of the pathological changes in blood lipids that is noted later) and reduced muscle building being the result.

Once the cycle ends and the user stops administering, the extra testosterone will slowly leave the body (time varies depending on the half-life of the drug used). However, oestrogen remains elevated for a slightly longer time so even if not used in the cycle, oestrogen management is generally required at this stage. Over time the user's natural hormone levels will hopefully return, though some form of Post-Cycle Therapy (PCT) is typically used to help this process happen. PCT is often used not only because it speeds recovery up, but because it increases the user's chances of recovering in the first place. The truth of the matter is that use can and very often does lead to permanent endocrine disruption in both sexes. Once the user's testosterone and oestrogen levels have returned to baseline the user is considered to have recovered and will often start to re-use in their next cycle.

Cycling can be psychologically difficult for many users. During the time they are on the drugs their muscles will not only grow faster, they will look harder and fuller, and they will be heavier due to water retention. At the same time the user will feel more aggressive in the gym, their strength will increase far faster than it usually would and they will typically lose fat (or gain far less than they should) due to nutrient partitioning favouring muscle tissue. In between cycles the user's testosterone will dramatically decrease before recovering (resulting in lethargy, low sex drive and poor mood) and all of these benefits will also go away. There is a reasonable chance of lost muscle mass between cycles, too, as testosterone signalling will be low to absent and therefore the lost muscle hardness and fullness will be exacerbated by genuine losses in size and strength. This is why, as we will come to, initial use often morphs into more prolonged and problematic self-administration.

At this point it would be useful for us to briefly cover how natural hormone production works so you are better able to conceptualise the impact that these drugs will have on the endocrine systems of both men and women.

23.9. Natural hormone production

The two systems primarily related to endocrine production are the HPT and HPO axes. The HPT axis is that found in men, involving the hypothalamus, pituitary gland and testes while the HPO is the same in women but involving the ovaries. You have already been introduced to the hypothalamus and pituitary in the module on stress and so are reasonably familiar with the overall pattern, but it should not surprise you to see that the specific signaller hormones involved with these axes are different to the ones seen in the HPA axis.

Here the hypothalamus secretes Gonadotropin Releasing Hormone (GnRH) into the portal blood which transports it to the pituitary gland. From here, Follicular Stimulating Hormone (FSH) is secreted into the bloodstream whereupon it binds on to and stimulates action within either the testes or ovaries to produce sperm, or eggs and oestrogen respectively. Leuteinising hormone (LH) is released from the pituitary at the same time. This stimulates testosterone production in men, while fluctuations in women trigger ovulation.

It shouldn't come to a surprise to you that these hormone levels are all fine-tuned to stay at a given level (which of course fluctuates in women), nor should it surprise you that this is mediated by a feedback loop which is therefore dramatically affected by steroid use. The loop works differently depending on the sex of the individual and so we will discuss these in turn, starting with the most common users.

In males the release of GnRh causes the release of FSH and LH. These trigger sperm production and testosterone within the testes. Receptors at both the hypothalamus and the pituitary monitor hormone levels, and as levels of GnRH, FSH and LH increase their production is subsequently reduced. Similarly, testosterone and estrogen both signal the hypothalamus to reduce secreted levels of GnRH.

If hormone levels become supraphysiological thanks to the administration of drugs, the signal from the hypothalamus and pituitary is reduced so significantly that endogenous hormone production ceases entirely. This is referred to as shutdown.

Not only do hypothalamic and pituitary receptors sense elevated testosterone levels and cease producing both GnRh and FSH/LH but also the testes release inhibins. These act locally on the testes themselves, signalling the leydig cells (the site of testosterone production) to stop working. As the testes are no longer producing hormone, the leydig cells start to atrophy and diminish in both size and number. This results in a reduction in testicular size and, if prolonged, this may never recover.

As hormone levels drop once steroid usage ceases, receptors sense the declining levels and the hypothalamus begins releasing GnRh again so the pituitary starts to release FSH/LH. Generally GnRh signalling and FSH/LH signalling return without complication, however if it doesn't it is known as secondary hypogonadism. If secondary hypogonadism is permanent then FSH and LH can be simulated by the drugs Human Menopausal Gonadotropin (HMG) and

LH, as well as the more common Human Chorionic Gonadotropin (HCG). HMG is arguably more effective as it mimics both LH and FSH while HCG only mimics LH, but the latter is far more widely available.

By far the more common is issue arising from steroid use is not secondary but primary hypogonadism with an absence in the return of testicular function despite proper FSH and LH production returning. An estimated 65% of long-term steroid users will eventually suffer this. Primary hypogonadism describes a situation where the leydig cells do not recover or are too badly damaged to produce testosterone. In this case the only option is TRT.

To try and avoid this permanent shutdown, most male users will run a course of other drugs, referred to collectively as PCT, after their cycle in order to try and restore natural function. We will return to this after exploring the effects of exogenous hormones on the female endocrine system.

In females as within males, GnRH results in LH and FSH production, however the action is now upon the ovaries. Females do produce testosterone (albeit to a far lesser degree than males). However only one quarter of a female's testosterone is produced within the ovaries. Another quarter is produced within the adrenal glands, and the remaining half is synthesised from other hormones within specific tissue. Regardless, all of these process operate with a negative feedback loop so as hormone levels elevate these processes are shut down, too. Of course the administration of testosterone results in some aromatisation in women and so oestrogen levels elevate, and this means that the ovaries reduce in size and due to the ceasing of FSH a female's menstrual cycle stops.

Not much more is known about the effects of steroids on the female endocrine system, and in fact it has long been believed that post-cycle females do not require any PCT as their body is used to very high and low hormone levels through the menstrual cycle. It was believed that the body would just pick up where it left off on the next cycle and hormone production would start up again.

In fact, for a large percentage of female users this is correct. However as female user numbers grow I am seeing an increase in females that don't recover and do require some chemical assistance to restart their hormone production. There is no set protocol for this but it would appear that 5 days of Clomiphrene Citrate (Clomid) or Tamoxifen Citrate (Nolvadex) use from day 2 to day 7 of the menstrual cycle is very effective at restoring hormone production. I am still working in this area, however, and it requires more research before I can say with any confidence that this is a viable treatment.

23.10. Post-Cycle Therapy (PCT)

PCT is a protocol of chemicals to rapidly restore natural testicular (and as you have seen, potentially ovarian) function. There is some debate over which PCT drugs are most effective and at which doses and duration, because as stated at the beginning of this module, steroid use for these purposes is by definition abuse and so very sparsely researched. Many cite Dr Michael Scally, a prominent endocrinologist who has worked with steroid abusers. His Programme for Wellness Restoration (PoWeR PCT) is often stated to be the most effective protocol, but even within the scant literature that exists on the topic this has its critics, and the lack of research in this area makes this a very debateable topic within the user community

There are three main drugs used regardless of the specifics of the protocol chosen. These are:

- **Human Chorionic Gonadotropin (HCG):** This mimics LH and helps restore Leydig cell numbers within the testes and therefore testicular mass

- **Tamoxifen Citrate (Nolvadex) is a Selective Estrogen Receptor Modulator (SERM):** This blocks the feedback receptors at the hypothalamus and the pituitary, making both of these glands think that hormone production is non-existent and so causing an increase in the release of GnRH and FSH/LH. As noted some users use this during their cycle to help minimise oestrogen-related side effects

- **Clomiphrene Citrate (Clomid) is another SERM:** This is also used this also helps with the blocking of the receptors at the hypothalamus and the pituitary gland

There is much debate as to whether both of these SERMS are required at the same time but at present it is common for both to be used because they have a slightly different mechanism of action. HCG is also debated hotly but has a great deal of anecdotal evidence as well as mechanistic reasoning behind its use.

The area of recovery is where we see the largest number of issues within steroid use, and it is estimated that 70% of all steroid users will eventually require hormone replacement therapy. It is difficult to really work out whether this figure is accurate because those who do require TRT are (evidently) able to get the drugs themselves without needing to go to a doctor and admit their participation in an activity that carries a lot of social stigma. This means that most people who need TRT will not have their usage recorded, but at the same time it means that many who do not need TRT didn't register as drug users in the first place. Regardless, TRT for under 25s on the NHS is currently higher than it has ever been and while many other things (obesity, etc.) could be to blame, it would be surprising if increased drug use in this demographic was entirely unrelated.

This problem just highlights the need for pre-use hormone testing in those who are still determined to use. Many users have no idea what their natural hormone levels are pre-usage, and the fact is that normal hormone levels vary dramatically between individuals. This means that even if they test post-PCT they have no idea as to whether they have returned to normal – many users rely on how they feel which is obviously not ideal.

To illustrate, the normal testosterone range in a male is 8.6-29nmol per litre of blood (nmol/l). Nmol means nanomoles, with a mole being the amount of a substance that contains 6x10^23 (6 with 23 zeroes) atoms, and a nanomole being one billionth of this (so 6^14 atoms). For testosterone this could also be stated as 280-1100 nanograms per decilitre of blood. Most people would not become symptomatic of low testosterone until 10nmol or less, so it is very possible for someone to not recover yet still subjectively feel fine. This often leads people to believe they have recovered when they have not and they start their next cycle early.

For example:

- User's natural levels are 25nmol/l

- At the end of his first cycle post-PCT and after a 12 week break he is at 19nmol/l. He feels fine and so starts again

- After his second cycle he is at 15nmol/l. He feels fine and so starts again

- After his third cycle he is at 12nmol/l. He feels fine and so starts again

- After his forth cycle, having run PCT and waited 12 weeks he is at 7nmol. He feels weak, lethargic and completely without a sex drive, so he tests and discovers that his testosterone levels are very low, and so may take a very long time to recover if indeed they ever do. Had he tested before his first cycle and again afterwards he would have seen that he had not recovered and so would have been more informed, hopefully leaving him to wait longer

This reduction in testosterone is not the only negative side effect of anabolic steroid usage.

23.11. Physical harms

For a long time, these have been downplayed by users and as they are very reluctant to admit usage to medical staff through fear of prejudice (which in many cases is quite well founded). Official records have backed up these claims of harmlessness – with many harms caused by steroids being attributed to something else by medical staff unaware of their patient's usage. Additionally, because there is a very positive view of steroids as 'harmless unless abused' in user communities and a large amount of denial on the part of the individual users themselves, it is very common for users to tell each other that they are not experiencing side effects even though they are, further promoting use and propagating the unfounded 'harmless' view.

With that said there is also an extreme prejudice against the drugs that is unfounded. The reputation steroids have as being killer drugs that are routinely responsible for organ failure, alongside overblown fears of 'roid rage' is dramatically overstated. Users note this and, because the mainstream fear of usage is not really warranted, they make the kneejerk decision to believe the opposite – that drugs cause harm. In fact, usage can be done somewhat safely with harm minimised, but in order to minimise harm it is important to know what it is you are trying to avoid.

It is self-evident that there are growing numbers of users experiencing health issues with numerous prominent bodybuilders and other athletes dying young, and with official records seeing a rise, too. The majority of problems arise because of mismanagement of the drugs themselves, with estrogen/progesterone/prolactin related ancillaries (drugs that mediate cosmetic side effects) being the most common drugs implicated. Issues include:

23.11.1. Infertility

The most prevalent and personally detrimental health impact is permanent endocrine shutdown and infertility. With regards to permanent shutdown this generally goes unrecognised in official records as users self-diagnose and medicate with unofficial TRT. They have access to the drug and the knowledge required to administer, and so begin self-treatment. Resultantly, this means it is never picked up by healthcare services and any official figures are likely to be unrealistic.

23.11.2.   Cardiac

Cardiac episodes have increased significantly in the past five years among top athletes, but prior to this period, cardiac incidents were rare. Through contact with users, many are reporting that the cardiac issues appear to be caused by unregulated blood lipids and arterial narrowing. However atomic remodelling, arrhythmias, hypertension, thrombosis, and erythrocytosis have all similarly increased in frequency. Anabolic steroids dysregulate blood lipids to a significant degree, and they can also cause hypertrophy of the heart – both are significant risk factors for heart attacks.

23.11.3.   Renal issues

These are becoming more common within the user groups. Current medical opinion within the NHS is that AAS use has no direct impact on the kidneys and that damage is caused by secondary actions of high blood pressure and increased body mass. Animal studies have suggested a causal link between the use of trenbolone and direct kidney damage, and there are a few case studies on acute kidney damage caused by this particular drug. As of this moment there is no clear relationship, but growing numbers of users are reporting renal issues which coincides with the popularisation of trenbolone itself. It is believed that it is only a matter of time before a link is confirmed. The number of AAS users reporting nephrotic syndrome has increased noticeably within the last 18 months.

23.11.4.   Liver incidents

These appear to be rare and though the vast majority of users show elevated Alanine (ALT) and Aspartate Transaminase (AST), respectively – two key markers of kidney health) whilst using, these tend to return to normal post-usage. Liver harm is primarily associated with oral steroid usage. Because these are ingested rather than injected into the muscle, and so the bloodstream, they must pass through the liver first. Over time this can cause toxic effects and ultimately liver damage.

Interestingly liver harm is far less than it otherwise would have been because users are often very aware of, and even exaggerate in conversation, the harms that come from oral steroid usage. As such oral usage is typically far more responsibly managed than is the usage of other drugs.

23.11.5.   Muscular and tendon injury

Though AAS have been shown to affect type 1 collagen, post-injury analysis has shown normal tendon integrity in users. It is believed that the effect of tendon integrity via weight training offsets any negative impact from AAS use. However, this does not consider the differential rates at which muscle to tendon strength increases. AAS rapidly increase muscular strength whilst tendon strength is somewhat slow in comparison. This strength imbalance does contribute to muscular/tendon injuries. However, hydration plays an equally significant role.

23.11.6.   Blood Born Viruses (BBV)

While there are a number of instances of users succumbing to BBV's (such as HIV) it is definitely the case that the risk of infection is far, far lower than estimated in official figures repeated on TV. This is because the current estimates for drug usage are likely to be dramatically lower than the true figure and so the reported cases of BBV actually make up a far smaller percentage of users than anticipated. Unlike users of other injectable drugs like heroin, steroid users almost never, if ever, share needles and current precautions (needle exchanges, online needle exchanges and awareness campaigns) are likely to be sufficient to continue minimising this risk.

23.11.7.   Hypothyroidism

The use of exogenous thyroid hormones such as T3 is common because this increases metabolic rate and so leads to elevated rates of fat loss. This can ultimately cause the same kind of shutdown as the hormone administration already discussed by disrupting normal production through a feedback loop. Many bodybuilders end up with permanent hypothyroidism requiring lifelong medication.

23.11.8.   Mental health

Without doubt, this is the biggest area for concern as more people with directly related steroid usage and mental health issues have come forward. The two are inextricably linked and in the author' view this is the most prevalent harm as a result of drug use outside of those linked to mismanagement. The main complexity in this area is assessing exactly how much is as a direct effect of the drug use, how much is a pre-existing issue that may have influenced the decision to use drugs and how much is environmentally based.

Most people enter the fitness world with a desire to change their physical fitness and their appearance. Prior to entering this environment there is usually dissatisfaction with these things, with individuals perceiving themselves as being unattractive or, in many cases 'only normal'. However once immersed in the environment of filters, photoshop and cleverly angled images their body image insecurities increase accordingly. Many report being more self-aware after getting into fitness than before, despite being objectively in better shape. This new-found pressure not only drives usage forward (as quite often they are presented with images that just are not possible naturally) but it increases insecurities (for example, why can't they look like that when others do?), and many report an increase in depressive episodes after becoming involved in the fitness world.

Studies have shown that AAS users have a greater frequency of depressive episodes than non-users that are taking part in exercise, and also a higher incident of anxiety (1).

Nandrolones have been shown to impact on neurochemicals, in particular GABA receptors. This neuropeptide has an impact not only on mood but also on a person's ability to form new memories. Many long-term nandrolone users report short-term memory issues with some being quite significant.

Anxiety is a common side effect of trenbolone, which is currently the highest selling steroid within the UK. Many users report severe anxiety issues and ongoing problems once usage has ceased. Users report losing their partners and their jobs and generally cease to function as a member of society whilst using trenbolone. Trenbolone is also tied to impaired sleep and increased aggression; while 'roid rage' is likely overstated this does not mean that it does not exist at all, and this drug in particular appears to be involved.

Furthermore, increasing numbers of people are becoming psychologically addicted. They suffer both physical and mental withdrawal issues and even prioritise their drug use over food, many eventually forming dependency on the drugs. Many feel they cannot maintain or progress without usage and so anxiety around body image prevents cessation. More and more users are staying on for prolonged periods of time; 3, 4 and even 5 years were commonplace during recent interviews with users. One individual had been using continuously for 10 years, and never used less than 1000mg per week. Being that a usage survey of 500 people in 2006 conducted by Parkinson and Evans (2) showed 80% were using between 500-2000mg per week, you should see that this was not a 'low maintenance dose'.

Overall it is worth bearing in mind that usage trends have seen a steady increase in doses, with the average user now reporting taking far more drugs than the professional bodybuilders of yesteryear.

23.12. The current situation with IPEDS within the UK today

Usage Image and Performance Enhancing Drugs (IPEDS) is growing at a steady rate. Trying to put an exact figure on the numbers using currently in the UK is difficult as steroid users are notoriously suspicious of any form of survey. There is a strong underlying suspicion of any official enquiry into user levels and many believe such evidence will result in the criminalisation of usage of the drug. It is this fear that actually keeps many from engaging with needle exchange services. This is compounded by many services having a lack of knowledge and having very little practical or useful information to provide to a user. Many extra services such as blood testing have been withdrawn due to lack of funding.

Many services lack proper training and as a result devalue the service they offer. Injectable consumables are relatively cheap so the ability to get these for free is not enough to attract users to these services. It is the author's observation that less than 20% of the users with whom he has spoken to engage with needle exchange services. Above we note that users are concerned about criminalisation; this is a common point of confusion and so it's useful to look at exactly where the legislation around steroids stands in the UK.

Anabolic steroids are controlled as class C substances under the Misuse of Drugs Act 1971 and scheduled under Schedule 4 Part II of the Misuse of Drugs Regulations 2001, both as named compounds (of which there are currently 69) and using a generic definition. The related drugs clenbuterol (a Q2-adrenergic agonist which helps burn fat), zeranol (nonsteroidal oestrogen), zilpaterol (another Q2-adrenergic agonist), somatotropin (growth hormone of human origin), somatrem (a synthetic analogue of human growth hormone), somatropin (synthetic human growth hormone), Human Chorionic Gonadotrophin (HCG) and Non-Human Chorionic

Gonadotrophin (NHCG) are also controlled. The various different forms, salts, and related preparations and products of all these substances are also controlled.

Anabolic steroids have limited legitimate use in the UK. Clinically, their main use is in the treatment of male hypogonadism (where patients fail to produce sufficient levels of testosterone). They are prescription only medicines and can only be lawfully sold or supplied in accordance with a prescription from an appropriate practitioner. It is legal to import and possess anabolic steroids, however, as long as they are intended for personal use and in the form of a non-medicinal product. However, the possession or import/export with intent to supply or manufacture is illegal unless authorised by a licence of the Secretary of State and could lead to 14 years in prison and an unlimited fine.

23.13. Drug availability

The availability of the drugs mentioned above are widespread are there are several routes of distribution to market:

Face to face: This is the traditional method and has remained quite consistent over the last 25 years. Typically transactions will occur in gyms (especially private-owned ones) as well as via meetups organised via apps like Whatsapp.

Websites: There are several websites offering IPEDs for sale. Many are fake sites set up with the sole intention of taking payment but having no intention of sending any product to the purchaser. There are some genuine sites but in general peoples' trust of these sites is very limited and as a result they are not a popular route for sourcing the drug.

Social media: Facebook has numerous selling and IPED related pages including some have even set up feedback pages for their customers. The clear majority of IPED sales are carried out via mobile phones although advertising may start via social media. Following the contact via phone, payment is made via PayPal or bank transfer and the product is sent and received by Royal Mail. This is by far the most popular distribution route of IPEDs to the end user.

More recently several underground laboratories have started to produce short video ads online. A recent example being for 'sphinx' (an underground brand) whereby the promoter altered the wording of the well-known Carlsberg advertisement, stating "if Carlsberg made steroids". These laboratories are starting to actively advertise and market their products in a way never seen before, using the anonymity of the internet to protect themselves.

23.14. Do we know just how much Is out there?

As mentioned above there are approximately 200 operating underground laboratories in the UK. Many of these are either 'homebrew' set ups with one individual, or otherwise small operations running with very low volume distribution rates. There are approximately 50 that distribute at a more noticeable volume.

These latter laboratories produce and distribute between 1000 and 5000 vials per week with the average purchase of between 5 and 8 vials. It is not unreasonable therefore to estimate that 100,000-200,000 vials of steroids are sold each week. This would equate to between 25,000 and 40,000 people purchasing steroids on a weekly basis. It is opined that this is an underestimation however, and the exact figures are extremely difficult to determine for obvious reasons. That said, it is clear that both production by these laboratories and consumption by users are far higher than many would assume.

23.15. The driving forces?

There are several factors pushing IPED usage forward, but the main two are a desire for easy and fast results, and unrealistic expectations coming from the media.

In general, modern society has promoted the idea of instant results with minimal effort. People want more leisure time and want to enjoy life more while still reaping the rewards of putting in hard work; which is reflected in marketing, social media and entertainment that promises instant gratification. There is also a desire to take a pill for every ill, with instant results expected from medicines, supplements and, drugs. The bottom line is that IPEDs (if they are the real thing) work, and they do so very, very well. A common thought process is "training and eating well are hard, so why bother when a pill or injection will do it for me".

Then, the surge in popularity of social media has exposed people to images of outrageous physiques more than any other technological advancement has before. Historically, body image pressures came from magazines but that was been tempered by the fact that many of those seen were professional models that most people understood were the exception rather than the rule. Now, people are exposed to so many people from so many walks of life with what they feel are better physiques than theirs. Males in particular are experiencing a level of body image pressure that they have never experienced before. Ironically, a large proportion of these images are enhanced via Photoshop filters and picture apps meaning the image portrayed is not realistic. However, many viewers are either not aware of this or chose not to accept it. The result is a distorted view on what is both achievable and normal.

Attempts to emulate these looks to gain social acceptance are destined to fail, resulting in frustration and feelings of inadequacy which drive individuals to ever more desperate measures and eventually drug use is considered. Programs like Geordie Shore and Love Island present an image of beautiful people having fun and enjoying a great life. They fail to inform the viewer that several of the participants are using IPEDs to achieve their looks.

As you can see, environment plays a significant role in driving use forward. Wales is generally regarded as having a very high per capita user level, for example, and a lot of this is fuelled by the gym culture within Wales (that and one of Britain's most successful bodybuilders being Welsh). Many of the gyms in Wales are local community based. What would be described in gym circles as 'spit and sawdust' places. These non-commercial gyms are a lot more open about usage with IPED uses not being a taboo as it is in many of the mainstream chain gyms. As a result, trainers are exposed to IPED use frequently and are therefore surrounded by people who they know are taking drugs, but who they can also see are in comparatively great shape. IPEDs are not regarded as secrets and their use is not seen as being a form of cheating, so discussion is open and it does not generally have negativity attached to it. Because of this use flourishes.

This means that we have a UK population that want to achieve a physique that is attractive, but who have surrounded themselves (at least online, which is the lens through which many view the world, or in their gym) with people who are far above the average. As such they view themselves as lesser. At the same time there is a desire to maintain a lifestyle that includes alcohol and junk food with minimal training, and a drug using community that dramatically downplays the side effects of usage. It is not all to surprising that many people are tempted to experiment and eventually use.

Even in open user circles, and on user pages, people are reluctant to openly admit arising issues and often maintain a façade of 'everything is great' whilst using these drugs (despite seeking support privately or just suffering in silence). For many, there is a reluctance to admit rising issues as they do not want to face the possibility of not using these drugs. Simply this is a case of burying their heads in the sand because they figure that if a person doesn't openly admit to having issues then no one is going to tell them to stop. During recent interviews, one known user who in the author's opinion was completely addicted, reported that he had not been for a blood test because he feared the results. There was no suggestion he had damaged himself but the result might mean he would have to stop and so he would rather not know.

This continual painting of steroids in the best light by the user community, at least in part as a result of excessively negative coverage by the media has led to a gross underestimation of their potential harms, further justifying usage as OK. Many cite TRT studies as support that steroids are not harmful, stating that they show testosterone to have many health benefits. These studies are not relevant in regard to supraphysiological doses but they are passed off as being so by several self-proclaimed steroid gurus.

One issue here is that even when research does exist, there is no research on multi-compound cycles despite these being something close to the norm (with users combining testosterone and nandrolone based anabolics with fat burners, HGH, insulin and all of the various ancillaries they need to manage side effects). The lack of evidence or clear knowledge pertaining to risks (beyond user trial and error) doesn't stop people going ahead however.

In general, the established, 'educated' user community regard IPED use as safe or at least that the risks are more manageable than they really are. They back this up with misquoted studies and a reluctance to admit any negative impact, while feeling that their healthy lifestyles and general fitness will offset the risks. It is difficult to determine exact figures on how much of a health risk usage poses especially in combination with an otherwise healthy lifestyle, but what is clear is that there are a growing number of people with health issues, particularly psychological ones including dependency.

For example, in the aforementioned interview the author did with an individual who, for all intents and purposes, is addicted to steroids and had been using nonstop for 10 years, this denial was clear. He was only 28 and since turning 18 he had not been below 1g of injectable steroids (many would consider this a high blasting dose). In fact, he often remained at 2g or above for literally years. He suffered physical and mental withdrawal issues if he reduced his dose to below 1g a week. He ran no oestrogen management and so had very advanced gynecomastia. There were periods in his usage when drugs were prioritised over food. Finally he had turned to illegal activity to fund his habit (selling the drugs). Though crime is not generally associated with the use of steroids like it is with other drugs, and in fact many users are what you might consider to be respectable in their everyday lives, the criminal act of selling them is very common. Many users turn to supply to fund their habits.

The response the current author got from the community upon releasing this interview was shocking in that the number of people that came forward with similar story or recognised something of themselves in the individual the author had interviewed was enormous.

Beyond the gym, usage within sports has grown. Historically it would have only been professionals that used to increase their performance, but now amateur sports are seeing the same. The author has spoken at length with ex-international athletes and according to their testimony, usage with field events and sprinters is common place with national team officials 'managing drug testing'. They spoke of several occasions where top flight athletes were instructed by coaches not to place in certain positions in races as they knew that position was going to be pulled for testing. Others were advised to be out or away from team training camps as testers were coming, and yet others said that known drug free athletes were tested more frequently than others "to make the numbers look good".

They stated that top flight athletes are managed to avoid drug failures. The motivation behind this is both political and financial. The embarrassment to a national team if a top athlete fails is huge but not only that, it is financially damaging. One has only look at the financial damage caused to USA cycling by Lance Armstrong's failed drug test to see how much of an impact it can have, both directly to the individual and team but also to the sport in general. Sponsors do not want to be associated with a drug cheat.

When asked about motivation, the athletes that were spoken to stated that a desire to be the best was a big driving factor, but also there was a financial aspect, especially for athletes in their twilight years where performance was starting to drop off – many viewed it as not having much to lose at this point. There was also team and national pressure and coach influence. On top of this the prevalence of usage amongst their fellow competitors was well known, so many adopt the attitude that in order to be competitive they have no choice. For example, many athletes state medical reasons for using certain things. Lots of asthma medications are stimulants that help with sprinting) but the athletes the author spoke to said that they did not believe their competitors and insisted that after 20 years of running an athlete doesn't just suddenly and conveniently get asthma in the run up to an event.

According to them there is a large scale cover up by sports bodies to protect their athletes from getting caught, more than any active attempt to prevent usage. The big motivator would appear to be financial: to avoid the loss of sponsorship. Within amateur sports there is a similar reflection particularly with regards to the attitude that everyone else is doing it and its necessary to be competitive. However, this obviously comes primarily from the competitors themselves.

Drug use is particularly strong in rugby, cycling and the use of calming drugs in such sports as archery and shooting, along with nootropics and ADHD medication in things like chess.

Outside of sports, the usage in middle aged and elderly individuals is, like for everyone else, driven by social imagery because there is pressure on all age groups. The older community are bombarded with imagery about staying young and being active, with advertisement campaigns by companies like Warner Leisure showing the older generation that being adventurous and very active is what they 'should be' doing while men become acutely aware of a loss of libido and virility. Many feel they are failing because they have less energy and 'get up and go' compared both to where they once were and what they see others their age group doing on TV. Often, they enquire about diminishing testosterone levels and are informed by their doctor that they are not eligible for TRT, as this is part of the natural aging process (while many women are given HRT, TRT is far less commonly prescribed). When they look up TRT on Google they find adverts selling steroids, and so the progression begins.

Though there is a stereotype of higher usage surrounding gay men this is not substantiated as far as the current author is aware. When people contact him, they disclose their usage but sexual preferences are not generally the topic of conversation! The author is aware of some of his clients being gay, but as there is no reason to assume a correlation between the two. He suspects motivations and usage rates will be similar to any other demographic.

The biggest driving factor across the board in the author's opinion is social pressure, including the flood of images posted on social media (the vast majority of which are not true reflections anyway). There is a definite influence from such shows as Geordie Shore and many young males try to emulate that look, feeling it will gain them success and popularity. Add into this a society that demands instant results and its 'a pill for every ill' approach to things and it is easy to see why there has been an increase in usage. Access to information regarding what to take is plentiful, as is access to the drugs. What is not readily available is access to information regarding preventive measures and safe practices. Some of the information regarded as safe practice is outdated and no longer relevant.

Irrelevant information provided by needle exchanges and GPs also does nothing but put users off from seeking advice and support from them in the future. Often when pushed, Harm Reduction workers and NHS staff cannot support their reasoning or advice with fact. This just turns users away from these services. Training within the NHS at a GP level is just not adequate enough to cope with the unique issues that users present with and there is a high level of prejudice towards users within the NHS. Again, this just drives users away from professional bodies into the realms of self-professed internet gurus and bro-science, thus increasing the risks they face. The current author has no doubt that over the next 5 years we are going to see a large increase in IPED related issues particularly linked to mental health.

23.16. How do the drugs differ?

As you can see from the section above that outlines some of the costs and prices of steroid manufacture and sale, there are a lot of different products available to users. One driving force behind the decision on the part of the user lies in the relative anabolic/androgenic balance as well as the basic hormone involved. There are slight differences between testosterone and nandrolone based steroids, meaning that combining the two allows a user to increase their dose (and so increasing the effects) while theoretically reducing their risk of incurring further side effects. The logic is somewhat similar to taking ibuprofen alongside paracetamol, rather than just taking a double dose of one of them.

Beyond that, however, drugs are classified by their esters and half-lives. A half-life is the amount of time that it takes for something to be 50% cleared from the body, a concept which plays on the fact that higher concentrations of things allow for a given amount to clear far faster than lower concentrations do. This means that (roughly speaking) it doesn't matter how high the concentration of something is, the half-life is the same. For example, caffeine is typically believed to have a half-life of up to 6 hours, which means that a 200mg caffeine tablet will act in the following manner (there will be some differences owing to absorption rate and first pass metabolism as well as binding to receptors etc., but this is illustrative of the point):

- **30 minutes after taking:** 200mg caffeine in the blood

- **6 hours and 30 minutes after taking:** 100mg caffeine in the blood

- **12 hours and 30 minutes after taking:** 50mg caffeine in the blood

This action is generally repeated around 7 times (meaning 1/128 of the original substance is still present) before the drug is considered to be cleared or 'spent'. A drug with a half-life of two days would therefore be 'spent' in 14 days.

Steroids in their pure form (commonly referred to as base or suspension) have a very short half-life of only a matter of hours. The half-life of testosterone suspension (testosterone mixed in alcohol without anything to slow release down) is generally listed as <24hrs, though anecdotally users claim an active windows of around 4 hours. This would mean the drug would need to be injected daily in order to stabilise hormone levels (if not more frequently) but as I'm sure you can appreciate this is impractical as well as painful (not to mention the risk of causing scarring in muscle tissue from repeated intramuscular injections) so drugs have esters added to them. An ester extends the half-life of the drug keeping blood levels stable for longer and reducing the injection frequency.

Esters are formed from carboxylic acids which effectively coat the hormone molecules. Enzymes within the blood decay this coating at a predetermined rate thus creating a stable release of the hormone. It is worth noting that esters have a molecular weight, so while 100mg of testosterone suspension contains 100mg of testosterone, 100mg of testosterone enanthate only contains 70mg of testosterone, with the ester taking up the rest of the space.

The following list shows the ester and its weight and subsequent impact on hormone content per 100mg. You don't need to memorise this, but it should offer an illustration:

- 100mg testosterone suspension (un-esterified testosterone): 100mg testosterone

- 100mg testosterone acetate: 83mg testosterone

- 100mg testosterone propionate: 80mg testosterone

- 100mg testosterone isocaproate: 72mg testosterone

- 100mg testosterone enanthate: 70mg testosterone

- 100mg testosterone cypionate: 69mg testosterone

- 100mg testosterone phenylpropionate: 66mg testosterone

- 100mg testosterone decanoate: 62mg testosterone

- 100mg testosterone undecanoate: 61mg testosterone

- 100mg trenbolone acetate: 87mg trenbolone

- 100mg trenbolone enanthate: 70mg trenbolone

- 100mg trenbolone hexahydrobenzylcarbonate: 70mg trenbolone

- 100mg nandrolone phenylpropionate: 67mg nandrolone

- 100mg nandrolone decanoate: 64mg nandrolone

- 100mg drostanolone propionate: 80mg drostanolone

- 100mg drostanolone enanthate: 70mg drostanolone

Each of these is chosen for different purposes. Users wanting to minimise injections will opt for longer half-lives, though this must be balanced by a greater difficulty in timing PCT. On the other hand those who need a fast clearance time (for example athletes who will be drug tested, or those wanting to minimise oestrogenic side effects such as water retention – competitive bodybuilders being a classic group) will opt for more frequent, faster cleared options. Below are the half-lives expected from different esters:

- Formate: 1.5 days

- Acetate: 3 days

- Propionate: 2 days

- Phenylpropionate: 4.5 days

- Butyrate: 6 days

- Valerate: 7.5 days

- Hexanoate: 9 days

- Caproate: 9 days

- Isocaproate: 9 days

- Heptanoate: 10.5 days

- Enanthate: 10.5 days

- Octanoate: 12 days

- Cypionate: 12 days

- Nonanoate: 13.5 days

- Decanoate: 15 days

- Undecanoate: 16.5 days

Looking to make this a little more clear-cut, below are some half-lives of common drugs used in the UK:

Half-life of commonly encountered injectables

- Deca-durabolin (nandrolone decanate): 14 days

- Equipoise: 14 days

- Finaject (trenbolone acetate): 3 days

- Primobolan (methenolone enanthate): 10.5 days

- Sustanon or omnadren: 15 to 18 days

- Testosterone cypionate: 12 days

- Testosterone enanthate: 10.5 days

- Testosterone propionate: 4.5 days

- Testosterone suspension: 1 day

- Winstrol (stanozolol) : 1 day

Oral steroids half-life

- Anadrol/anapolan50 (oxymetholone): 8 to 9 hours

- Anavar (oxandrolone): 9 hours

- Dianabol (methandrostenolone, methandienone): 4.5 to 6 hours

- Methyltestosterone: 4 days

- Winstrol (stanozolol): 9 hours

Ancillaries half-life

- Arimidex: 3 days

- Clenbuterol: 1.5 days

- Clomid: 5 days

- Cytadren: 6 hours

- Ephedrine: 6 hours

- T3: 10 hours

As you can see there is a huge disparity between the active half-lives of various drugs, and so the dosing of them must be properly thought out by the user. Unfortunately, most users will not do this (or at least won't do it properly) and so mis-dosing and uneven hormonal levels are common. Most users are also not aware of the impact of esterification on the concentration of the drugs they are using, and so they will count a 250mg dose of something as being 250mg of an active substance, when it isn't. This can cause mis-dosing and mismanagement if a user is no longer able to purchase one drug and instead opts for another with a different ester.

23.17. What are the most common drugs

It would now be useful to give you an overview of the most common drugs, what they do, why users would choose them and how they are typically run. All of the below drugs are prone to the harmful side effects listed above, and so we will only list the desired effects here – just remember that none of the below are exempt. Accompanying this module are some fact sheets located in your online portal – please look to those for further information.

Drug: Testosterone Enanthate
Type: Injectable steroid
Half-life: 10.5 days

Usual dosage: Ranges from 250mg upwards to the extreme of 5g per week. The most common range is 500mg to 1.5g.

Desired effects: Increased muscle mass. This is the stereotypical 'base drug' that almost every steroid protocol will utilise.

Drug: Dianabol
Type: Oral steroid
Half-life: 4.5-6 hrs

Usual dosage: 30-100mg.

Desired effects: Increased strength and size both through genuine anabolic effects and extreme amounts of water retention. Gains are lesser than injectables because liver toxicity limits dosing.

Drug: Nandrolone Decanoate (often referred to as Deca)
Type: Injectable steroid
Half-life: 14 days

Usual dosage: Ranges from 300mg upwards to the extreme of 5g or even more. The most common range is similar to testosterone 600mg to 1.5g.

Desired effects: Thanks to a far higher anabolic to androgenic ratio it is a fantastic muscle builder that is also useful for promoting collagen synthesis (so it aids with joint and tendon issues). This has a high binding affinity to androgen receptors, however, so natural production is strongly shut down often leading to impotence and a loss of sex drive even while on cycle.

Drug: Anavar
Type: Oral steroid
Half-life: 9hrs

Usual dosage: 10-100mg.

Desired effects: Increased size but primarily increased strength and 'hardening'. It has a low aromatising effect, so water bloat is minimal to zero. It slightly upregulates thyroid hormone production, promoting fat loss. Virilisation is very low, making this popular amongst females.

Drug: Clenbuterol
Type: Oral fat burner
Half-life: 1.5 days

Usual dosage: 80-160mcg.

Desired effects: Because it activates beta-2-adrenergic receptors in fat tissue it promotes fat burning. Also causes shakes and cramping.

Drug: Winstrol
Type: Oral (though can be injectable)
Half-life: 9hrs

Usual dosage: 10-100mg.

Desired effects: This drug is non-aromatising so no water retention presents, and it also lowers progesterone so can help remove excess water gained from other drugs. This is used to help 'dry' a physique out for competition, but this can cause joint pain.

Drug: Trenbolone Acetate
Type: Injectable
Half-life: 3 days

Usual dosage: 25mg eod for females up to 200mg eod for males.

Desired effects: Strength and muscle size without aromatisation. This is promoted as the best drug for 'aesthetic' gains and it also garners huge strength improvements thanks to effects on the motor nervous system. Psychological and physical side effects are far more prominent than they are with almost all other drugs.

Drug: DNP
Type: Oral fat burner
Half-life: 36hrs (though there is some dispute over this)

Usual dosage: 100-400mg daily. This is, however, dangerous at any dose.

Desired effects: Rapid fat loss.

Concerns with this drug are far greater than many of the others. DNP works by interrupting the proton gradient in mitochondria. You will recall that the electron transport chain ultimately works similarly to a dam, with electrons being pushed through a protein channel and generating ATP. As this is interrupted the body cannot produce ATP and instead energy is wasted in huge amounts through heat. This is self-evidently very effective for fat loss as the body loses the ability to properly perform respiration and so must burn through its stores.

Unfortunately, the body has no defence against this action and no chemical will neutralise it nor will it 'flush it out'. This means that someone taking a dose that is too high risks overheating without any means of cooling down and this can lead to death. Unfortunately, because this is a drug taken daily with a relatively long half-life this means that doses overlap and so serum levels rapidly increase over the course of a few days, meaning that dosing is very difficult. This is also coupled with the fact that all DNP available is made and dosed in underground laboratories where mistakes in dosing can happen.

Generally, it is used in short blasts of a few days at a time or lower dose long-term. At short duration the lowest recorded death was caused by a dose of 4mg/kg/bw, and long-term usage the lowest dose causing death was at 1mg/kg/bw.

On top of these drugs there is one more form that have risen to popularity in recent years – Selective Androgen Receptor Modulators (SARMS). We will briefly cover these now, explaining what they are, what they are purported to do and how they compare to traditional IPEDs in terms of both desired and side effects.

23.18. Selective Androgen Receptor Modulators (SARMS)

These were developed to try and create a purely anabolic substance that did not meaningfully interrupt natural hormone production, so all of the benefits and none of the risks. At the time of writing none have actually achieved this, with many still having some androgenic effects on the prostate yet many are commercially available. There are two kinds, steroidal and non-steroidal with the non-steroidal version being increasingly popular. These work by binding on to specifically chosen androgen receptors and causing effects (such as muscle building and accelerated fat loss) but because they aren't hormones and because they aren't binding to other receptors such as those in the HTP axis, they do not readily cause shut down (though this is possible with higher doses).

They are oral and are classed as research compounds, so sale of them is legal if purchased for research, though no enforcement of that is placed on the retailer (meaning you can buy them over the counter in many instances). They are often a gateway drug to steroid use because although they are generally well tolerated with few if any side effects, they give low to moderate results when compared with their steroid counterparts, meaning that temptation to take 'the next step' is high. As mentioned, a high dose can also lead to testicular atrophy or female virilisation because as yet the products have not quite achieved the precision selectivity that manufacturers are aiming for.

23.19. Summary

So, what's the big attraction to steroids or any performance enhancing drug? Well the bottom line is they work (as long as they are the real thing). Steroids will increase your muscle mass, fat burners will reduce fat, and they will both allow this to happen far faster and more successfully (muscle will come with less fat gain and fat loss will have little to zero muscle loss alongside it). In an ideal situation if you chose to use any of these drugs you would do so when you had exhausted the natural alternatives and make sure that other factors had already been optimised, such as diet and training.

Unfortunately, that isn't how the real world works and for many, the effectiveness of these drugs means that they are viewed not as an aid but as a shortcut – minimising necessary amounts of work. It is often quoted that there is steroid use and steroid abuse. Now technically all steroid use outside of a medical setting is abuse but within the user community this statement stands very well.

It is possible to use steroids and have a relatively healthy relationship with them, with minimal impacts on your health. In fact, I have seen drug usage transform lives in a positive way. For example:

- People with low testosterone levels who have been rejected by the medical profession because they are considered to be at the very bottom end of what can be considered 'normal', often suffer all the symptoms of low hormones. They can be depressed and unable to maintain relationships, jobs and suffering with very low self-esteem. I have seen individuals such as this self-prescribe TRT and become a different person with a totally new lease on life

- The current author has seen fat burners and steroids help turn a morbidly obese, shy, shell of a man into a flourishing healthy human being

- Even when these drugs are taken for performance enhancement the current author has incredible success stories in athletes and bodybuilders that have come with zero negative consequences

But in all these cases the key factor was that the drugs were secondary to diet and exercise rather than the main focus, and harm prevention was of primary concern. Users had regular bloodwork, spent significant time cycling off the drugs after a proper PCT (other than the first example), and they did not ignore side effects. On top of that the correct ancillary drugs were used to limit the negative effects of excessive oestrogen build-up, and perhaps more importantly they slept well and avoided alcohol, smoking and recreational drugs.

Sadly, it is becoming increasingly more common that the drugs are the focus and that no due diligence is paid because the perception amongst users is that steroid use is 'no big deal'. People don't educate themselves on the effects of these drugs, they have poor diet and an unhealthy lifestyle, and they partake in cross polymer drug use that only compounds the problem.

Psychological dependence is very common. Users are scared to stop using, resulting in either very long-term use or very high dose use. This results in an exacerbation of all of the potential side effects and there is evidence emerging to support withdrawal and addiction.

Mental health problems are a concern amongst users, with depression and usage being highly correlated, and certain drugs altering neurochemical secretions resulting in memory loss. A growing number of users are turning to products like Cannabidiol (CBD) oil in an effort to combat steroid induced anxiety and historically cannabis smoking has been prevalent, yet when the proposal of reducing doses is suggest all manner of excuses are presented.

Can steroids be used safely? The answer to that depends on your definition of 'safe' but they can definitely be managed effectively. Probably the biggest long-term health risk with steroids is because of the cardiovascular effects. All steroids increase LDL (particularly orals) and some decrease HDL this results in an unhealthy cholesterol balance that in time will lead to plaque build-up on the artery walls. Couple with this the fact that steroids increase the red blood cell count and blood pressure as well, as causing hypertrophy and stiffening of cardiac tissue and it's not surprising that heart attacks are a significant risk. A big problem here is that the heart attack may come 10-20 years after usage and so (combined with a low level of self-reporting) the link has always been hard to draw, but as more and more bodybuilders are falling prey to heart attacks the link is becoming clearer.

High blood pressure can also cause damage to the kidneys. Acne is common both because of unstable hormone levels resembling that of teen years, and because of heavy metal contaminants in the steroids themselves. There are also issues like inflamed cranial fluid though it is rare, it has been reported via steroid use and a variety of other physical risks.

Finally, infertility is very, very common.

So with all this in mind can these drugs be run safely? As already noted, 'safe' is a relative term but with education and information risks can be minimised. In order to minimise risks you need to know what going on, so testing is extremely important. Users knowing their hormone and blood markers prior to usage is essential as you then have a record of what is normal for that individual. After that there are a few essential steps that must be taken:

- **Users should prioritise their training and diet before drug use.** The more efficient the first two are the less of the third they will have to use

- **Time off is essential.** Completing a proper PCT and then taking time of all drugs minimises risk of infertility and allows for unstable blood lipids etc. to return to normal. Continued use will guarantee testicular function issues and increase side effect risk

- **A healthy lifestyle should always be adopted.** While using a potentially harmful compound you do not want to be adding more stress to the body via other drug use, alcohol, poor sleep, smoking or sedentariness

- **A healthy diet** can also help your blood lipid markers as well as aiding in the normal detoxification of contaminants contained within the products themselves

- **Protective supplements have some anecdotal support.** Products like taurourso-deoxycholic acid (a bile acid that may help support the liver) and Saw Palmento for the prostate are common, while some companies also produce all in one supplements, specifically designed for cycle support. These are often questionable or completely unsupported by the literature, however, so a user should not expect to be able to use these to counteract any harms that may otherwise have befallen them

Ultimately there are no guarantees. These are potentially addictive drugs with serious side effects and so the recommendation that we will always stand by is that their use should be avoided as a rule of thumb. Risking your health for the sake of body composition or gym performance does not represent a good risk:reward ratio. With that being said, a sensible user can minimise risks provided they initiate usage having taken the necessary precautions (proper physical testing) and provided they do so without the major negative self-beliefs which would predispose them to addiction-like behaviours.

23.20. References

1. Piacentino, D., Kotzalidis, G., Casale, A., Aromatario, M., Pomara, C., Girardi, P. and Sani, G. (2015). Anabolic-androgenic Steroid use and Psychopathology in Athletes. A Systematic Review. Current Neuropharmacology, 13(1), pp.101-121.

2. PARKINSON, A. and EVANS, N. (2006). Anabolic Androgenic Steroids. Medicine & Science in Sports & Exercise, 38(4), pp.644-651.

3. Wedinos.org. (2018). *WEDINOS - Welsh Emerging Drugs & Identification of Novel Substances Project*. [online] Available at: http://www.wedinos.org/ [Accessed 27 Jan. 2018].

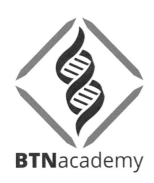

BTNacademy

MODULE 24

TEAM SPORTS NUTRITION

24. MODULE 24: TEAM SPORTS NUTRITION

24.1. Module aims

- To explain the importance of nutritional interventions for team sports

- To advise clients around the different energy pathways used for different disciplines.

- To provide macronutrient recommendations

- To offer in and off-season advice – what changes?

- To advise around setting up a week of nutrition, with training and a game

- To speak on the subconscious desire for aesthetics in sports, and around fat loss or muscle gain in and off-season

- To discuss the drinking culture in sports

24.2. Key principles from module 23

The last module covered IPEDS, image and performance enhancing drugs. This is a complex topic with a lot of nuance, but you learned:

- There are a huge number of drug users in the UK, with those numbers increasing for various reasons

- The motivations for use differ amongst users

- There are a vast array of drugs with different anabolic:androgenic profiles, half-lives and esters

- Use is not criminal, though manufacture and sale is

- Users may use continually at a low dose (TRT), on and off, or continuously at varying doses

- There are a significant number of risks including permanent shutdown of testosterone function and CVD

- Harms can be reduced but not eliminated, and whether use can be safe depends entirely on the user's definition of 'safe'

24.3. Introduction to team sports nutrition

When we think about nutrition coaching or fitness in general, it seems almost odd to say it but we often forget about what is potentially the largest sporting demographic in our industry – team sport athletes. Though powerlifting and physique sports dominate the world of online fitness, it is by far rugby players, football players, hockey players, basketball players and competitors from almost countless other disciplines which make up the majority of athletic individuals in the general population. Therefore knowing how to manage the nutrition of this kind of client will allow you to potentially work with a far larger number of people.

Team Sport players are not only greater in number than physique or strength athletes, their needs also make them far more complex. When working with a team sport player our recommendations must take into consideration the sport in which the individual takes part in, the position or role that they play and how much game-time they get vs. bench time, what part of the season it is at any given time, the frequency of games vs. training and the stresses of travelling to games (along with the inconvenience this brings to controlling nutrition). On top of this, while a bodybuilder or powerlifter require only one facet of fitness, a rugby player or lacrosse athlete needs to optimise speed, power, endurance, strength and agility all at once. As such their training can be far more demanding. All of this means that we must perform a constant juggling act between optimising performance with adequate fuel, managing recovery as effectively as possible, and keeping bodyweight and body composition relatively even, because both weight gain and loss might be uniquely damaging.

A large factor that we must consider on top of the nuts and bolts of a diet for a team sports athlete is the fact that they will often (even at the elite level) live in a very different environment to that of a client looking only to optimise health and performance in an individual sport or in the gym. A team sport player is a part of a certain culture particular to the sport they play and will have some peer pressure to deal with – this may or may not be conducive to what would be considered 'perfect health'. For example, one famous study found that (because it is normalised and even encouraged), US college athletes were far more likely to drink heavily and drink often compared to students not involved in athletics (1).

This is by no means the case for 100% of athletes, but it certainly isn't the exception. Often a coach will find a certain amount of ambivalence felt towards eating to optimise health and performance – that is, after a game an athlete may know that eating a healthy and balanced meal with adequate protein and carbohydrate is important, but what they will actually want to do is go to the local with the rest of the team and have the beer and burger meal deal, or head to the club house for pints and pies.

It is here that you should be able to see the importance of a client centred approach and a respect for a client's autonomy. It is very unlikely that any resistance from you is going to change the behaviour of this client, and in fact it might damage your relationship going forward if you are insistent. It's also prudent to remember the big picture and consider the importance (or lack thereof) of this relatively small part of the client's week.

Again – this is a generalisation and as with all similar statements, exceptions exist. Treat each client as the individual that they are, and you can't go too far wrong.

24.4.   Build a Foundation

A client who plays a team sport will typically have a far higher energy need than a client who trains solely for body composition, assuming similar NEAT. While a strength athlete (which is what the latter are, in effect) only really needs to consider 3-5 sessions per week of roughly one hour, team sports athletes have a more demanding regime. They have to consider any gym work they do (and there should be some), sports specific training and drills, and then games which can be, generally, considered the most intense and demanding session of the week. Training will span both anaerobic and aerobic work and depending on the sport and position in question, there may also be some sessions more closely resembling that of an endurance athlete.

All of this adds up to a large calorie burn, and so the first port of call should be to match this. Unwanted weight loss or gain can both cause trouble, with increased weight adding additional strain on the joints and cardiovascular system as well as impairing weight:power ratio and so slowing the player down. On the other hand, a study in the New Zealand Journal of Sports Medicine (2) highlights that significant undereating in athletes can result in:

- Decreased sport performance effects due to decreased muscle strength, glycogen stores, concentration, coordination and training responses, and increased irritability

- Increased negative health consequences, such as injury due to fatigue, loss of lean tissue, and poor nutrient intakes, including essential nutrients, due to limited food intake

- Increased risk of disordered eating behaviours due to severe energy restriction

- Increased risk of dehydration, especially if the diet is ketogenic

- Increased emotional distress due to hunger, fatigue, and stress related to following an energy-restricted diet

While weight loss is often a goal for team sports athletes (2) and something we will discuss later, suffice it to say for now that most athletes would do well to either lose weight very slowly or to maintain it during heavy training periods, such as in-season.

Calculating a team sport athlete's energy requirement is the same as it would be for anyone else and so we would ask you to refer back to the module on calculating TDEE to find out the process for doing this if you aren't sure. With that being said it is very important to carefully consider the variable nature of team sports calorie requirements and so keeping a closer eye on weight fluctuations and perceived daily energy will more than likely be necessary. While training days are likely to stay the same week to week, a client might find themselves spending a month drilling set pieces and ball work, then the following month working on acceleration and top sprinting speed.

Clearly these two modalities have differing energy requirements and so the client is likely to need more or fewer calories (primarily from carbohydrate as you will see) at different times depending on what goes on. It is for this reason that there is likely to be a significant amount of adjustment needed week to week and calorie estimations (unless the player is able to find out what the whole season of training is going to look like) are typically made reactively rather than proactively. That is, a client will be asked to eat more by their coach because last week was tough, rather than being able to make that change prior to the increased intensity.

One means of combatting this is to rely on some degree of subjectivity and provide a client with a calorie range to aim within – perhaps you calculate a female lacrosse player's maintenance to be somewhere around 2800kcals, factoring in two strength training sessions, three sports training sessions and one game per week alongside a reasonable amount of NEAT. This client could be given the target of 2700-3100kcals per day, affording her the option of eating a little more if she feels that training has been particularly tough, or sticking with a lower intake for a typical day. The client would then rely on their own experience of their training and resultant hunger to make informed decisions (promoting autonomy and self-reliance). If the client starts to gain unwanted weight, the solution would then simply be to converse with them and come to a better understanding of when it is and is not entirely appropriate to shoot for the higher end of the range.

It's also important to discuss this from the other angle. Many sports performance athletes desire weight loss (2) and may under report or intentionally under estimate their activity levels and thus undereat as a means of keeping their body weight down. Be vigilant and always double check what a client tells you by comparing weight shifts, energy and performance with calorie intake.

24.5.   Macronutrient intake

Once the athlete's daily energy needs are calculated, we need to figure out how that energy will be best distributed between the macronutrients. Typically, the way you recommend a client distributes their macronutrients will depend on the nature of their sport and the overall training that they do. While it would be nice to be able to give a blanket recommendation for team sports, we cannot do this as the needs of one athlete will differ from another.

Furthermore, there is a potential need to increase carbohydrate intake during certain periods and counteract this by reducing it at others to leave a net average – but we will discuss this in the next section once total intake is worked out. Before we discuss carbohydrate needs, we will go over protein because recommendations do differ between sports independently of calorie intake.

When working with a client we need to be aware of the form of training in which they are engaging throughout the week. A rugby player who requires more physical size and strength than a footballer (soccer player) will be doing a lot more strength training and also be using that strength a lot more during games, meaning his protein need will be higher. Although there is a strength component to football, more so for central defenders and some attacking players than other positions, football is mostly about skill, speed, agility and endurance, meaning that the strength training component of their week will be significantly diminished in comparison.

These are just two sports used as examples, you need to figure out the total training load of the sport and adjust protein intake accordingly using a rough sliding scale. The International Society of Sports Nutrition recommends 1.4-2g of protein per kg/bw per day in order to properly build and maintain muscle mass in athletes, with endurance-based athletes requiring something closer to the lower end and strength athletes being closer to the higher end (3). This is similar to the recommendations stated earlier, of 1.6-2.2g/kg/bw, highlighted in a review by Helms et al (4). A slightly higher figure of up to 3.1g/kg of lean body mass (total mass minus bodyfat percentage) may be needed during times of energy restriction (3) but we will return to this later.

The 1.4-1.6 range is likely to be adequate for the majority of team sports where additional strength training is a small component of the weekly regimen, provided they are at energy balance. This not only increases our ease of managing nutrition, it will allow for a higher intake of valuable carbohydrate as fuel. Most footballers, field hockey players, basketball players, baseball players, table tennis players, cricketers and volleyball players fall into this category.

Next would be athletes who perform a small to moderate amount of strength training and/or take part in a particularly physically demanding sport, either in terms of hard contact or in terms of massive energy output. Though these athletes may not seek hypertrophy or dramatic strength improvements as a general part of their game, protein intake needs to be sufficient to reduce muscle loss as much as possible and help recovery in general. A somewhat higher intake, closer to 1.6-1.8g/kg/bw would be apt for these individuals – think lacrosse players, water polo players, those taking part in highland games, those who do roller derby or even some footballers who approach the game from a much more physical standpoint.

Finally, we have athletes such as rugby players, American football players or similar who's sport not only involves being athletic, but strong too. These athletes will be training on the pitch and playing in games but will be accompanying this with a progressive and structured resistance training routine which must be accounted for. An intake of 1.6-2.2g/kg/bw is a good range for these individuals, and as noted you may even take this a little higher during a dieting phase.

After this is accounted for we need to distribute the rest of the athlete's caloric allowance and generally speaking you start with assigning calories over to fat. The reason we opt for fat first is because fat intake is necessary for proper bodily function and so avoiding an excessively low intake is important. For example, a paper in the Journal of Sports Science and Medicine (5) highlighted that undernutrition in athletes was associated with:

- Joint inflammation
- Soft tissue inflammation
- Systemic inflammation
- Airway inflammation
- Increased sympathetic nervous system response to high intensity exercise

All of the above have been improved by increasing dietary fat in some research (5). Other research also indicates a potential link between dietary fat intake and serum sex hormone levels (5) and so it's safe to say that a minimum amount would ideally be adhered to. Finally, very low-fat diets have a notoriously poor rate of adherence, probably due to the interaction between dietary fat and various gut hormones as explained when we discussed digestion, and the mouthfeel/taste that dietary fat provides.

With that being said, an increased fat intake within a given calorie intake is not likely to improve sports performance because, as discussed in the endurance training module, the anaerobic activity involved with almost all sporting activities physiologically cannot be fuelled by fatty acids. Together this means that a minimum amount of fat intake is needed, but that fat shouldn't be emphasised.

A 'moderate' intake of dietary fat is typically described as 20-35% of total calorie intake (5) with the UK RNI being <35% (6). Most athletes would do well to opt for the lower end of this range, but personal preference and adherence will always be the final factor. You could speak to the client and ask what kinds of foods they prefer, and judge from that whether they tend to opt for higher or lower fat foods and you could then make recommendations accordingly.

Carbohydrates are the last macronutrient to consider. They should, simply, make up 'the rest' of a sportsperson's intake. The figure at the end may seem relatively high, but that is due to athletes generally having high energy needs overall. So to sum up:

- **Calorie intake:** Approximately maintenance accounting for activity. Opt for a range that allows the client to eat a little more if activity is especially high on some days and monitor weight closely

- **Protein intake:** 1.4-2.2g/kg/bw, depending on the demands of the sport and the client preference

- **Fat intake:** 20-35% of intake, scaled upwards with calorie needs and preference

- **Carbohydrate intake:** The remaining calories

Of course, in order to actually implement that you need a few things in place, namely:

- A client that tracks calories

- A client that tracks macronutrients

- A client that is willing and able to do and adhere to both every day

It is unlikely that you will find many individuals like that, at least initially. A pragmatic solution is to simply ask the client to monitor protein and calories, opting for higher calorie whole foods in order to make up their total intake. You can then monitor a client's macronutrient intake and work with them, making suggestions, to bring it closer to the theoretical ideal over time if this is required. A number of alternatives have been suggested in the module on nutritional tracking, so please refer back to that if needs be.

Of course, it's not all about calories and macronutrients.

24.6. Building good habits

Contrary to what many fitness professionals will assume, the average team sports player will hold many, if not all, of the same beliefs and attitudes towards eating healthily that the rest of the general public do. In fact, in many instances their dietary habits are worse rather than better thanks to a combination of not really being interested (as most people aren't), existing in a culture that can promote poor choices, and being able to 'get away with it' in terms of not gaining excess weight thanks to a high energy output. This means that lean proteins and vegetables typically aren't the focal point of a team sport athlete's diet.

A team sport athlete has a high energy output, but they are also subject to a great deal of stress and pressure during games, they spend a lot of time outdoors in all weathers, and they can spend a lot of nights in hotel rooms when travelling, depending on their level. From another viewpoint, a lot of team sports players will be university students who survive on very little sleep and spend a lot of time around other people in close quarters – all of this means that their immune system needs to be running on all cylinders to avoid illness.

This is a perfect opportunity to utilise what you know about self-determination theory and motivational interviewing. Rather than dictating to the client that lean proteins and vegetables must be eaten, you are able to raise their awareness of the impact that these foods have on their ability to recover from activity and, perhaps most salient, their ability to avoid missing out due to illness. As with any client progress will more than likely need to be made slowly as habits improve but adding a portion of vegetables here and working to increase protein there, can over time lead to a far better dietary intake. It will take a long time to change the culture surrounding the team and its attitude towards eating, but by opting to make small changes and appeal to their personal values, you're able to gradually make progress.

A final note here is to consider fibre. We have previously recommended roughly 10-15g of fibre per 1000kcals of intake, which falls roughly in line with the UK guideline of 30g per day (6) but allows some room for scaling up and down according to individual intake. This should, however, be taken only for 'typical' intakes, and we propose a theoretical maximum intake of around 50g per day. Going beyond this is likely to lead to GI distress and constipation. As such, athletes with a very high calorie need may need to opt for lower fibre carbohydrate sources at times.

24.7.   Setting up the week

A team sport athlete's week can typically be viewed as a cycle. The beginning of the week is a recovery phase, leading into a training/preparatory phase and culminating in a weekend game. This is, of course, assuming one game per week (higher frequencies will be briefly covered momentarily).

Assuming this one game per week frequency, it is often pertinent to carbohydrate cycle somewhat in order to maximise glycogen availability come game-day. This need not be a hugely complex process, and in fact making the difference between the day(s) before a game and the days afterwards too large can have fairly obvious consequences to recovery. Doing this by increasing carbohydrate hugely the day before a competition as a 'carb load' has been commonplace within many sports for a long time, but in reality, this 'bolus dose' approach is mistaken.

When we bolus dose ingest nutrients, your digestion process simply slows down to compensate (7). What this means is that often, eating a lot of carbohydrates in a large meal the day before a game just leaves you bloated on game day. Consider instead opting to slightly skew carbohydrate intake a little higher for the 24-48 hours before a game instead, much like you would for an endurance athlete who was going to compete for 90 minutes.

Typically, athletes are told to eat a large, carbohydrate filled breakfast before a game in the theory that it will improve performance. What usually happens in reality is the client feels dreadful and bloated, which of course affects performance negatively. To counteract this, increasing carbohydrates the day before game day will allow the athlete to eat a normal breakfast before playing and go into it without a huge bowl of oats on their stomach – a tactic which proves even more useful if the athlete is on the road at away games and finds it impossible to get to a good meal. This also allows the client to increase their food intake after the game, potentially making that pie and pint a little easier to fit into their requirements.

To do this, follow a basic carbohydrate cycling approach by taking total carbohydrate intake as a weekly target and 'skewing' it around the week. An example may be.

Client needs an average of 500g carbohydrates per day, so 3500kcal per week.

- Monday: Off – 500g carbohydrates
- Tuesday: Light training and gym work – 400g carbohydrates
- Wednesday: Off – 400g carbohydrates
- Thursday: Heavier training session – 400g carbohydrates
- Friday: Gym work – 600g carbohydrates
- Saturday: Off or skills-based session – 600g carbohydrates
- Sunday: Game – 600g carbohydrates

This slight variation is realistically only going to be necessary for very competitive athletes. A typical Sunday league player may simply reduce calories by roughly 100kcal per day Monday-Saturday and then 'spend' those calories on game day. Remember, there is no perfect setup and your approach must be tailored to the client at hand. All we ask you to keep in mind are principles.

24.8. Game day considerations

Our job is to help the client find a way to fuel themselves adequately for training and recovery during the week, then deliver them to the coach on game-day ready to go. This means we need to discuss strategies for during game day with the client, including what would help before, during and after the competition itself.

Critically, we can work with our client to create a pre-game meal (usually breakfast) which meets their needs. It should contain protein, carbohydrates and some fats but may be lower fibre to avoid bloating. That said we should go with client preference to a significant degree because realistically, provided the total carbohydrate intake for the rest of the week has been as it should be, your client will be more or less as fuelled for performance as they could be by the time they wake up. Pre-exercise ingestion of carbohydrate has not been shown to strongly influence performance provided glycogen storage is adequate (8) and therefore the purpose of this meal is more to make them feel ready rather than to actually prepare them physiologically. If there is a large gap between breakfast and playing, a small carbohydrate and protein feeding 60-90 minutes ahead of the starting whistle may be useful to provide immediately usable blood glucose and amino acids.

Once this has been done, your recommendations are going to be mostly in terms of what the athlete will do. On game-day, emotions are high, team spirit takes over decisions, and peer pressure is massive. Additionally, you want them to focus more on trying to win than trying to get a certain meal eaten and understanding their priorities is important. With all of the best intentions in the world, it is unlikely that an athlete is going to adhere to the healthiest diet possible, so we need to respect that and make recommendations where we feel they will not be ignored. We know that prior to a game we can usually influence the client's food, so make sure that they consume a meal which will make them feel good, that they are hydrated, and they take something with them to consume before starting to warm up (as noted above).

During the match itself, consuming carbohydrate at a rate of around 30-60g per hour of exercise in a drink that provides 6-8g per ml (an isotonic drink) is likely the ideal (8) as this has been shown to improve performance in prolonged exercise situation, so utilising a sports drink (either powdered or pre-made) or even a standard piece of fruit at half time alongside water is a great recommendation to make.

After the game, again we need to think about what the client will do and make compromises. If your client will come off the pitch and mix up a recovery drink or protein shake then that's fantastic; if they are going to quickly change and go to eat a balanced meal elsewhere that's even better. However, oftentimes it could be a few hours before your client gets home or gets some solid food, and even when they do it's likely to be suboptimal, so settle for what they **will** do. Chocolate milk, a protein bar or something else sweet is a good bet for most.

After that, we need to work with what we have in front of us. Some clients will be easy and will finish the game then head home. In this case, the advice is the same as always – consume your macronutrients in a layout which suits you, using mostly whole foods. If not, there may be a point where you just have to ask your client to consume their recovery drink and then be sensible, as post-game junk food and alcohol is part and parcel of a lot of team sports, and your client may not be happy if you ask them to miss out. This is not to mention, as noted already on the course, a couple of pints isn't likely to hamper recovery or health to a meaningful degree.

If the client regularly overindulges post-game and this leads to unwanted weight gain, tackle it then and discuss options. Perhaps they limit alcohol a little more, or they cut calories from other days to compensate. Don't be afraid to discuss this with the client but do so in a manner that communicates the fact you won't change things the client doesn't feel need to be changed. Remember, we cannot influence a person unless our recommendations align with their values, beliefs, needs and wants.

24.9.   Recovery tactics after games

Various recovery strategies are utilised by many sportspeople in order to maximise their performance day to day. It's great to be your best during a game, but if that means that you are incapacitated for 2-3 days afterwards that will affect training and ultimately effect performance as the season goes on. These are some simple recovery tactics which could be recommended to your athletes:

- **Consume an adequate amount of food.** If a client is undereating the rest of these recommendations aren't going to really make a difference. Interestingly, this can even be a problem for the real 'post-match party' people, because while it's not all that healthy, having 5 pints and a burger after your game and then going to sleep might mean your client has under eaten when the whole day is taken into account. Bear this in mind if your client regularly feels lethargic the following day

- **Maximise sleep.** Like any other client, sleep is vitally important to team athletes. Bear in mind that they may be spending time sleeping on coaches or in shared hotel rooms, so investing in an eye mask and some earplugs could be a very good idea

- **Regular sports massage.** Most teams have an in-house physio but don't take this for granted. Weekly massage should be seen as a good approach to looking after the muscles and contributing to maintaining flexibility (many athletes are poor at sticking to their mobility routines despite a coach or physios wishes)

- **Self-myo-fascial release using a foam roller, stick roller and hockey ball between massages can be useful.** While evidence for this is not concrete regarding injury reduction, it does appear to assist with pre-exercise mobility and post-exercise recovery rates (9)

- **Consider ice baths and even NSAIDS if game frequency is acutely high.** Anti-inflammatories or ice baths can reduce delayed onset muscle soreness, but they can also blunt the adaptive response to training (10,11), meaning that you will stop being so sore quicker, but at the expense of progression. This sounds bad but consider that some athletes may have numerous games 72 hours apart during busy periods of the season but they need to be completely recovered and ready for each. The ultimate decision is the client's, but it would not be the end of the world to utilise these methods for a few difficult weeks at the end of the season, in the context of a full year of training

- **Supplements may be considered.** Further details are provided in the Foundation Academy manual, but beta alanine, creatine, caffeine, and beetroot extract (sport depending) all timed and dosed appropriately may be useful ergogenic aids alongside any regular supplementation such as fish oil and multi-vitamins that an athlete may take

- **General stress management, as always, cannot be overlooked either.** An amateur athlete has to deal with the stresses of their sport but also of their real life too. Don't forget that your 110kg number 8 client may also own a business and have a child to feed when they get home. Balancing life and training while minimising required effort around food are two big factors in longevity for many

24.10. Season timing and other considerations

Unlike other clients who are mostly interested in strength or body composition improvements, the needs of a team sports player may differ depending on the time of year and, critically, you aren't the only professional who is helping them achieve their best. Your client will have a coach, potentially a strength and conditioning coach (if you are working with them online and not training them in a gym) and maybe a physio. This could be viewed as a 'too many cooks spoil the broth' problem, but it's best to instead view it as a multi-disciplinary team of experts, who take care of different aspects of your client's progress.

The important thing here is that you will need to work with these other professionals and show them respect by communicating and never stepping on toes. You need to display a united front for your client or you will lose your coach:client relationship very quickly. By explaining your methods and involvement to the coach you will get their buy in as well as your client's. You can use the team physio to help keep on top of potential injuries and even request training and season schedules from their coach so you can plan ahead, as alluded to above.

During heavy training periods such as pre-season your client may need more food. During times where games are more densely packed due to re-scheduled matches or cup games you will need to focus more on recovery than anything else, and during the off-season there is a potential for calorie needs to go either up or down depending on what your client wants to do in their downtime.

Always bear in mind that the time of season, the scheduling of games and the periodisation of your client's training will change their needs and this may be completely out of your control. All you can do is plan for it by knowing ahead of time when energy needs are going to change and adjusting carbohydrate intake accordingly. You can also use these periods to alter the body composition of your athlete, which we'll cover in more detail in the next section. If the training schedule cannot be acquired, at least try to locate a list of regular fixtures and tournament games so you can find out their game frequency. The rest will need to be played by ear – communication with your client will be critical.

24.11. Body composition improvements as an athlete (2)

So far, we have discussed team athletes in terms of performance but we can't ignore that these clients are people too, which means that body composition is likely to be a secondary (perhaps even primary) concern to them for personal reasons unrelated to the sport (2). Of course, fat loss goals may not be unrelated – football, for example, is a game that generally caters toward a leaner individual and while some players will achieve this leanness effortlessly this will not be the case for all, and so we can say that weight loss athletes will fall into two camps:

- Clients that are overweight for their sport

- Clients that are lean but who wish to lose weight for aesthetic reasons

Both situations may require a different approach.

Most sports have an 'ideal fat range' which rarely stretches low enough for someone to have visible abs. Being too lean as a sportsman means that you will have less stored energy for use later in games, you'll have less insulation for playing in cold conditions and, at the most basic level, you'll have less padding for resisting contact with the floor, walls or other players.

Those who are too lean are more injury prone and more likely to become exhausted in the last important minutes of a game (2). Here a discussion needs to be had which is honest and realistic – the fat loss goal needs to be achievable, realistic and also conducive to performance. A client may want to lose additional weight beyond that needed for their chosen activity despite the risks associated with doing so, and that is their decision to make, but you should still make them aware of the facts. This will be especially important for younger clients.

Likewise, there may be times when an athlete wants to gain weight. This can realistically be done with a lot more flexibility, as weight gain should not really impact performance so long as you take things at the usually expected slow rate to minimise fat gain. The only consideration with weight gain is the training which you may need to implement.

24.12. Fat loss with an athlete

The considerations here are numerous, outside of what has already been covered with the lower limits of leanness. Let's not forget that the fitness industry has largely forgotten what fitness actually is, and often correlates extremely low body fat levels with extreme fitness. This is not the case at all, and more often than not the physique sports are the antithesis of fitness in every way.

When looking to help a team sports client lose fat we need to first assess how far the client has to go. For someone who is currently carrying a lot more fat than they should for general health, let alone performance, the process should be relatively painless, at least initially. With that said, a slower and more patient approach is still likely to be preferable if the client has a heavy training regimen. Reducing calories by roughly 10-15% on average over the week is a good rule of thumb in-season, because more rapid fat loss may lead to the decrements in performance listed in an earlier section. Aiming for a slower 0.5-1% of fat loss per week is a good place to be.

During off-season you have more wiggle room because training strain is going to be reduced. During off-season your client has no games to worry about and usually no formal training, either. They will probably maintain resistance training and some amount of basic endurance training but the point of off-season is to recover and take some time off. This affords the perfect chance to increase their fat loss rate to closer to 1.5% of bodyweight per week.

Easy places to start instigating nutritional changes include post-game indulgences (raising awareness of the impact this has may help the client make better choices – two pints rather than five) and mid-game sports drinks. It would also be prudent to 'stack' carbohydrates pre and post-training and playing, rather than distributing them during the day, as this could theoretically improve performance and recovery while allowing restriction to occur at other, low activity times (2).

24.13. Weight gain with an athlete

If your athlete wants to gain muscle, two things will need to happen. They will need to increase training volume and increase calories. They may also need to increase protein if they fell into a more endurance-based bracket. This would seem like it could be done at any time, but we need to be mindful of total training volume and total recovery capacity. Even with the best sleep, most optimal nutrition and perfect stress environment, there is only so much an athlete can recover from. If the overall training regime is demanding already, muscle hypertrophy will be impaired even with the best approach because allostatic load will eventually overcome anyone.

For many amateur athletes this will not be a huge issue, as the training they do will not be that demanding. Their results will be slower than they ordinarily would be if they only lifted weights, rested and ate, but they won't be completely absent. If your client is training a lot and they want to add yet more training in order to build muscle, it is your responsibility to explain to them that this might not work as well as they would hope, and in fact could hamper recovery from everything else they do. The client will need to make a value judgement and decide whether they want to wait until later in the year or reduce their sport-specific training in order to chase a secondary goal at the expense of performance.

Overtraining in its truest sense is very rare and probably not an issue for most clients we will encounter (it represents a systemic form of 'burnout' that is hard to actually achieve), but overreaching recovery capacity and being overcome by excessive allostatic load is more common than you would think. If a client perpetually trains beyond their recovery capacity, you can in fact cause regression rather than progression, leave them exhausted, with reduced immunity and generally burned out.

It is for this reason that muscle gain is best saved for the off-season when total training load is reduced and you can focus on squat strength without worrying about having tired legs on Sunday. During the season, stick to 1-3 resistance training sessions with low to moderate volume. This is not to say that progression shouldn't be the focus nor is it to say that hypertrophy can't or won't happen even on this reduced volume. However utilising something like the strong lifts training program for in-season to maximise athletic performance and reduce total fatigue when recovery capacity is needed elsewhere; then ramping up volume during the off-season to build muscle mass, is the best approach you can take for most sports. Some clients will not accept this and will want to do more, but provided you advise low-ish volume and a manageable frequency, you should find a compromise.

24.14. Coaching a team/club

If you happen to be working in a team environment as their nutritionist, all the same rules apply. You are going to want to improve the team's hydration, calorie intake, timing, supplement use, and much more. What is important in this environment is analysing all the variables and see what small changes you can make over time. Understand the team/club's financial and time constraints, the levels the players are at, and the amount of buy in from the team and players. You know how to coach a team player, you just need to see where you can affect small elements of change over time with the team, having constant feedback loops with the players and staff regarding the changes you are making.

Communication will make or break your success as a team nutritionist, you have to work as a unit, and if at any point you start implementing things on your own accord it will upset the apple cart. Remember you're not just working with 20+ autonomous individuals, you're working with the collective team too, and so you have to respect their culture and gain permission before you start to do what they will see as "telling them what to do". Slow and incremental change is the way to go in most instances and producing written content for the team to read so they are aware of why you're advising what you are is a great start.

Consider bringing in a hydration strategy work sheet for all players, a simple explanation of macronutrients and their uses, suggest where to buy supplements that would benefit them, give them some recipe ideas, put on a few evening seminars for the players and spouses (it's always important to create the right home environment, and family is included in that), ensure they are getting their pre and post-game meals correct, give them a stress fact sheet and ways to improve stress factors in their lifestyle, all simple ideas you can do over time to educate the team and players in a group environment.

Never enter a team environment and try to change too much at once. You are the outsider and will have to earn the respect of the club and players regardless of your background. Indeed, it can take years to change a team's culture. Below are some suggested tactics to increase your likelihood of success in this environment:

- Spend time building rapport

- Bond with difficult players to make sure there is no one undermining your efforts from within the tight-knit circle

- Bond with the team decision makers (as this will pass down into the team quicker as they follow their lead)

- Show them you are human and not just a coach/authority figure – get involved in social events with players

- Keep your advice real – always bearing in mind the reality of the environment you are in and the dynamics

- Understand the rituals and history of the club or the sport

- Appreciate any difficult dynamics the club currently has so you can be sensitive where needed about certain situations

- Show humility to players with difficult situations – if you show you care you will earn respect quicker

- Get involved in game day and show you have an interest in the club and player's success and that your role isn't just a 'job' for you

- Be effective at working with the rest of the coaching staff, never cause friction, always find ways to work with the staff, not against them

- Consider training with them in a fitness session to show you are getting involved (this will work in some clubs and environments, but not others, so think about this point carefully)

- Learn about other teams and players in the leagues so you have relevant talking points about the competition, including you in the clubs' weekly focus and dynamics

- Above all, appreciate that you're not the expert dictating things to the team, you're a part of a system and you need to work alongside the other parts. As soon as you see yourself as above the rest, they will stop listening to you

24.15. Summary

As you can see, a team sport athlete must be treated somewhat differently to the standard client. Their needs are varied and specific, and this means that client:coach communication channels must be kept as open as possible, as well as cultivating a strong relationship with the other exercise professionals who assist your client.

Meet total energy needs, ensure macronutrient intake is tailored to the sport, the position, the time of season and enforce good habits with your athletes. Beyond that your focus as a coach should be on keeping their recovery as top priority while 'coaching around' the various social barriers that your client will encounter, always looking to work with the environment rather than against it and respect the client's wishes, guiding and advising rather than dictating and instructing.

24.16. References

1. Ford, J. (2007). Alcohol Use among College Students: A Comparison of Athletes and Nonathletes. Substance Use & Misuse, 42(9), pp.1367-1377.

2. Manore, M. (2015). Weight Management for Athletes and Active Individuals: A Brief Review. Sports Medicine, 45(S1), pp.83-92.

3. Jäger, R., Kerksick, C., Campbell, B., Cribb, P., Wells, S., Skwiat, T., Purpura, M., Ziegenfuss, T., Ferrando, A., Arent, S., Smith-Ryan, A., Stout, J., Arciero, P., Ormsbee, M., Taylor, L., Wilborn, C., Kalman, D., Kreider, R., Willoughby, D., Hoffman, J., Krzykowski, J. and Antonio, J. (2017). International Society of Sports Nutrition Position Stand: protein and exercise. Journal of the International Society of Sports Nutrition, 14(1).

4. Morton, R., Murphy, K., McKellar, S., Schoenfeld, B., Henselmans, M., Helms, E., Aragon, A., Devries, M., Banfield, L., Krieger, J. and Phillips, S. (2017). A systematic review, meta-analysis and meta-regression of the effect of protein supplementation on resistance training-induced gains in muscle mass and strength in healthy adults. British Journal of Sports Medicine, pp.bjsports-2017-097608.

5. Lowery, L. (2004). Dietary Fat and Sports Nutrition: A Primer. Journal of Sports Science and Medicine, 3(3), pp.106-117.

6. Public Health England (2016). Government Dietary Recommendations. [online] London. Available at: https://assets.publishing.service.gov.uk/government/uploads/system/uploads/attachment_data/file/618167/government_dietary_recommendations.pdf [Accessed 11 May 2018].

7. Calbet, J. and MacLean, D. (1997). Role of caloric content on gastric emptying in humans. 489(Pt2), pp.553-559.

8. Kerksick, C., Harvey, T., Stout, J., Campbell, B., Wilborn, C., Kreider, R., Kalman, D., Ziegenfuss, T., Lopez, H., Landis, J., Ivy, J. and Antonio, J. (2008). International Society of Sports Nutrition position stand: Nutrient timing. Journal of the International Society of Sports Nutrition, 5(1), p.17.

9. Cheatham, S., Kolber, M., Cain, M. and Lee, M. (2018). The effects of self-myofascial release using a foam roll or roller massager on joint range of motion, muscle recovery, and performance: a systematic review. International Journal of Sports Physical Therapy, 10(6), pp.827-838.

10. Schoenfeld, B. (2012). The Use of Nonsteroidal Anti-Inflammatory Drugs for Exercise-Induced Muscle Damage. Sports Medicine, 42(12), pp.1017-1028.

11. Roberts, L., Raastad, T., Markworth, J., Figueiredo, V., Egner, I., Shield, A., Cameron-Smith, D., Coombes, J. and Peake, J. (2015). Post-exercise cold water immersion attenuates acute anabolic signalling and long-term adaptations in muscle to strength training. The Journal of Physiology, 593(18), pp.4285-4301.

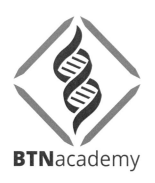

MODULE 25

NUTRITION FOR BODYBUILDING PREP

25.   MODULE 25: NUTRITION FOR BODYBUILDING PREP

25.1.   Module aims

- To explain what is involved in competition prep, and what the end goals should be

- To describe the process by which those goals are attained up until peak week, including nutrition and training

- To explain how to assess the client for the proper protocol

- To advise around refeeds during the process

- To give a clear run down of peak week and competition day in terms of nutrition and training

- To provide information around the psychological impacts of competition prep

- To offer information around the post-prep period, and what to do in order to ensure the proper physiological and psychological recovery

25.2.   Key principles from module 24

The last module covered the varied and interesting role of coaching a team sports athlete, or indeed the team as a whole. It's a fantastic niche to work in that affords access to a large part of the market, but of course some unique things need to be taken into consideration. You learned:

- Team sports athletes will need different things depending on their sport, position, and standing within the team (do they start, or are they on the bench?). Things will also vary between different parts of the year, and so careful periodisation is necessary

- Carbohydrate loading may be necessary ahead of games. The easiest way to manage this, however, is to skew carbohydrates and calories slightly more towards game days if the client is tracking these things

- You don't just need to work with the person/team, but with the culture of the sport too. It can take a long time to create change and so rapport/communication is probably more a part of this job than any other in nutrition

- Any changes to body composition are far easier to do in the off-season. Fat loss in-season must be slow while strength gains at this time may be very difficult to do, due to training loads

25.3.   Introduction to nutrition for bodybuilding prep

Throughout this course so far when we have spoken about fat loss it has been in the context of improving health first and foremost. While we have briefly discussed fat loss in terms of improving physical appearance in some places, the former aim has been our focus simply because it is the reason that the vast majority of people will want to lose weight when they come to a coach or trainer. However, it is not the case that fat loss is done for the sole purpose of improving health or attractiveness, in some instances it is done in the name of sport or competition.

In the next module we will discuss weight loss for strength sports and fighting athletes who will need to make weight, and it should be known that similar principles to those discussed in those modules will apply to a number of other sports, such as synchronised swimming, horse racing, dancing and a number of gymnastic events. For now, however, we will be paying attention to bodybuilding, physique, bikini and fitness photoshoot contest preparation (referred to as 'prep').

In this module we will explore what prep is and what the desired outcome is, before discussing the various things an athlete needs to have in place in order to achieve this goal. From there we will then look at the post-dieting period, during which recovery and a return to a normal state of health is sought after. We will rely as much as possible on direct, high quality research and data but you should know that the totality of available literature pertaining to contest prep is relatively scant, and so in places we will be utilising published case studies. These can be an incredibly useful form of research, but they do have obvious limitations that we ask you to consider when reading. Namely, it's not always the case that individual cases will illustrate generalisable principles that apply to every single individual. With that being said, the patterns highlighted are generally considered universal.

We will also not be exploring in great depth one area of prep that is valuable to consider in light of what has been discussed so far, and that is the reasons that someone would want to compete in a bodybuilding or physique competition in the first place. Suffice it to say that reasons will include:

- Competitiveness
- Ticking something off a bucket list
- Genuine passion for the chosen sport
- The opportunity for sponsorship and industry involvement
- To create marketing materials based upon photos in a given condition
- To create social media pictures for likes and personal validation
- A personal challenge and task to overcome
- Peer pressure in certain gyms/social circles
- Body dysmorphia
- Eating disorders

Needless to say some of these reasons are arguably more positive than others. It would be unethical for a coach to work with someone who has a diagnosed eating disorder in the manner stated during this module, and the same goes for someone with diagnosed body dysmorphia.

This is not so straight forward, however, because one could very easily argue that bodybuilding, physique and even bikini competitions (the distinction will be explained momentarily) necessitate the behaviours associated with both kinds of mental health problems in order to win. Someone looking in a mirror multiple times per day, restricting their food in order to lose large amounts of weight (despite this causing low energy and mood as well as endocrine disruption), and fixating on the relationship between their food intake and how they look in the mirror, could be a bodybuilder or someone with a disorder – the outcomes and motivations may differ but the actions are the same.

It's also not unusual for competitors to display a pathological poor relationship with food and self-image during contest prep, especially towards the end, even when these were not there before. One study (1) found that 46% of male bodybuilders engaged in post-show binge eating and 81.5% reported a preoccupation with food – both of these are indicative of disordered eating. This means that, to an extent, the development of poorer psychological wellbeing is normal and almost expected during this process even in healthy individuals. It will not happen to all, of course, but it does occur and a coach needs to look out for it.

Each individual, and indeed every prep that a given individual does needs to be considered a standalone case. It's safe to say that starting a prep phase with someone who is already nervous around or restricting food, or someone who attaches their entire self-worth on what they see in the mirror (or what they think they do) is a bad idea. These issues are likely to crop up at some time during prep even if they aren't there at the start, and this is why a trusting and honest relationship with clients is so important. We will discuss this topic more in a later section.

To close this introductory section, we ask you to look back at the list of potential reasons (note that it's not exhaustive) and see if you can see which are intrinsic or extrinsic motivations. Take a minute to think about which of these is more likely to lead to a real drive to succeed when hunger is high and energy very low, and which is likely to lead to 'falling off the wagon' and binging, or simply hating the entire process. If an individual is not likely to have their why lining up with their actions, they may have the grit to continue, but seeing as they will get no real satisfaction from the end result, what is the point?

Talk sincerely to any client who is approaching you to do a competition or photoshoot and ask them why. Discuss where the idea came from and how long they've had it, and make sure they understand completely the drawbacks and negatives as well as the positives so they can make an informed decision. Once they have done that they are ready to go.

But go where?

25.4. What is contest prep?

Contest prep is the process of dieting down to extremely low levels of bodyfat (with levels of 'extreme-ness' being dictated by your particular sport) whilst maintaining a large degree of lean body mass (again, relative to the sport). This is done in order to compete on stage, posing alongside fellow competitors to be given scores by a panel of judges. The process typically involves a combination of caloric restriction and resistance training alongside an appropriate amount of cardiovascular training, culminating in a week or so of 'peaking', which is a short-term strategy to maximise appearance on the day. Typically, a diet will last somewhere between 8 and 30 weeks, with around 24 being the average in most instances.

This can be viewed more or less like an extreme diet, with the goal being bodyfat levels often far lower than what could be considered healthy or even attractive. You will then peak in order to show off your condition before regaining weight and (hopefully) health. This last part is important and will form a significant part of this module. As you will see there are some significant health ramifications for being at an extremely low level of bodyfat, both psychologically and physiologically, not to mention the increased risk of muscle loss that occurs as calories get so low.

In fact, most competitors maintain their peak conditions for 1-2 days before regaining weight and will only achieve this shape a few times per year at most. Most competitors also don't compete year to year, with it being relatively normal to take one or more years off at a time between competitions in order to build more muscle and make progress between prep phases.

The un-healthiness of the final outcome is one reason why those who have been through competition prep will often describe it as such a difficult process. You are pushing your body to do things which it ultimately does not want to do, and therefore it will fight back. As you have learned numerous times already, when dieting you will be hungry and lethargic. However, when the diet end goal is the extreme leanness associated with physique sports you are also likely to be cold, irritable, sexually dysfunctional and even to get 'prep brain' where basic communication is poor and you slur or mix up your words. These will be explored more in a later section.

25.5.   How lean are we talking?

The condition that constitutes 'stage ready' will be different from sport to sport, though with this said it's very rare to see a natural competitor get too lean for their particular competition and be docked points because of it. It does happen, but this is generally speaking a better prospect than not being lean enough. If you are too lean, you can pose differently and use your tanning products carefully to mask it, but there's no way to fake leanness that you have not achieved. If you are wondering if you're lean enough but also concerned you may overshoot your best condition, risk overshooting rather than falling short.

The amount of leanness required for each contest will be different depending on the judges and the specific federation. The criteria for each is largely subjective and based upon the judges' present, but generally speaking they will be along the lines of the following.

Bikini: Stylish hair and facial beauty, a balanced, symmetrical and 'complete' physique which is firm and lean, but not overly muscular or lean. Competitors must be free of muscle separation or striations, while also being free of cellulite or other skin blemishes. In recent years there has been a heavy focus on well-developed and 'full' gluteal development.

Men's physique: Muscular and lean, but not to the same level as bodybuilding; meaning the 'dry' look bodybuilders shoot for is not seen as a positive. The physique must be balanced and complete, with a small waist, prominent abs and obvious V-taper, though leg development is less important owing to the 'board shorts' worn on stage. The overall package is considered, including facial aesthetics, grooming, the shorts you wear and your overall 'male fitness model' quality, which again is a subjective term making it hard to really know what to go for.

This is currently the most popular category at bodybuilding shows, likely because the individuals do not have to diet to the same unhealthy and unattractive level that bodybuilders do, and also the level of musculature is achievable to a far broader set of people (either because naturals do not have to have a freakish ability to build muscle, or because drug assisted athletes do not require such a vast concoction of different compounds).

Fit body: Symmetry is important with the upper and lower body being in proportion. Muscle tone is the key, with a larger amount of muscular separation than would be expected in bikini, but still without the musculature, striations, capped deltoids and 'hard look' associated with bodybuilding.

Bodybuilding: Get as big as you can and as lean as you can, whilst maintaining some semblance of balance.

There are many other categories, but these are the main ones.

For this module we will focus on bodybuilding specifically as the demands are the highest. For other categories the general approach would be the same, but a smaller amount of muscle gain would be needed in the off-season and prep would generally start a little closer to competition. Bear this in mind as you read on. As a final note, we will also be exclusively considering natural or drug free prep, rather than prep assisted by IPEDS.

25.6.   When are you ready?

We all know one or two people who seem to be 'ready for stage' year-round either in our gyms or on social media. You may see them with legs like road maps and washboard abs, but the truth is that if this person really does look like that year-round, they are more than likely 6-8 weeks away from actually being in competition shape. Modern gym lighting (especially gym bathroom lighting) is generally really good because gyms know their audience and lighting can make a huge difference to your appearance. One of the worst mistakes competitors make is to judge their physique in great lighting, after working out.

Lighting on stage is notoriously, and intentionally bad. It's there to show off your flaws and make the judging easier, and as such this is the kind of setting you should really seek out. This is why, generally, people will look way better in their prep photos than they will on stage photos. True bodybuilding stage condition looks freakish in person; like a walking anatomy chart, and if bodybuilding is your goal, suffice it to say you should be able to see striations in your glutes as standard. For the other categories the actual end-goal leanness will be less severe, and it would pay off hugely to familiarise yourself thoroughly with the typical look of on-stage competitors before you start planning your diet.

One thing that often holds people back from achieving true stage conditioning is their preconceived ideas surrounding bodyweight. A competitor on stage will be a lot lighter than they look, because that level of leanness isn't something we are used to seeing and so we don't have a good mental idea of what bodyweights are typical. A good model for your maximum on-stage bodyweight is the rough guideline proposed by Martin Berkhan of Leangains.com, which is to take your height in centimetres and minus 100, to give a reasonable estimate of your maximum bodyweight in stage condition. There will be individual variation of course, depending on genetics and bone structure, but this is a pretty sobering thought for people expecting to be 100kg lean at average height.

This shouldn't be something which you find disheartening, however. Leanness has the ability to give the impression of size, and it's often said that the fastest way to look like you gained 5kg of muscle is to lose 5kg of fat. This becomes very apparent when you see a 75kg competitor on stage who looks like he would be 90kg or more. We must also remember, that your final bodyweight makes no difference when it comes to placing.

Ultimately the condition that you need to be in, in order to compete, is dictated by your particular category. The best option is to go to shows and find pictures of competitors and compare yourself to them in poor lighting. Having another person do the same is a valuable guard against either over or underestimating your readiness, too. Be open to criticism here – too many competitors turn up out of shape because they refuse to believe friends and coaches who tell them they aren't ready to compete.

Now we have a rough idea of where we want to go, we can look at the first part of the journey to get there, the basics.

25.7.   Prep: The basics

As mentioned, competition prep involves a prolonged diet to an extremely low bodyfat level, while maintaining as much muscle mass as possible. The first thing you need to consider is just how long you believe it will take to get you to there, because starting a diet too late will leave you missing the mark, while starting far too early risks exacerbating the negative effects of dieting.

As discussed in an earlier module, the typically recommended rate of weight loss is roughly 0.5-1.5% of bodyweight per week and this holds for the initial stages of competition prep. However, the actual rate of loss needs to be dictated by current leanness because increased leanness amplifies risk of muscle loss during hypocaloric conditions (2, 3) and so your deficit must decrease in severity as you get closer to show day. Realistically this means you may lose 1-1.5% of your bodyweight for the first few weeks but then decrease this to around 0.25% per week in the final stretch.

A good way to estimate the amount of time it will take you to get ready is to take your current bodyfat level and the goal bodyfat level; then double the difference between these two to get a number of weeks, allowing for a 0.5% bodyweight loss per week. Realistically this is going to be far slower than you really need to go, but it's going to maximise muscle retention and perhaps just as importantly, it allows for various slip ups and plateaus without adding too much pressure.

A female at 26% bodyfat looking to compete at 15% would therefore take 22 weeks to prepare for a contest.

As discussed already on the Academy, it is very difficult to accurately ascertain your bodyfat percentage and so this calculation will by necessity include a reasonable amount of estimation. Unless a DXA scan is available (or BODPOD) it is likely that the best way to do this is by eye or, if you know how to use them, callipers. By the time you are able to coach a physique competitor you should have a reasonable idea of what various different levels of bodyfat look like. While it is incredibly unlikely that you would get it right (people store fat differently, and even if they didn't this approach is very prone to human error), this method at least gives you something of a starting point. Because the method of calculating how many weeks your diet should be has a wide margin of error, this is an acceptable approach for starting to plan your tactics.

Beyond that, the nutritional methodology taken in order to prepare for a contest is a relatively straightforward one – at least up until the last few weeks. It follows more or less the same advice given for any other dieting approach, but with a slightly more rigid style relating to certain factors. Note that this should still not be prescriptive, and the client's views should be considered but for this goal nutrition must be more precise; we are looking for a specific short-term outcome. The first thing to consider is caloric intake.

25.8. Calories

A deficit sufficient to lead to 1.5-0.5% of bodyweight lost per week is required, and as the client gets leaner their loss rate will need to decrease. An observational study noted that this is in fact the opposite of what usually happens (4) with competitors dropping calories further and further towards the end of their diet and losing more lean body mass as a consequence. No hard and fast rule exists for the exact points at which the calorie deficit should be lessened, but as a rule of thumb, a competitor could diet at a rate of around 1% bodyfat per week until they were around 4-5% bodyfat away from their ideal condition, and then rate of loss should be slowed.

Adaptive thermogenesis will need to be taken into account here, and it may be the case that no calorie adjustment is needed at all (or indeed calories need to be dropped further, even though a slowing of weight loss is desired). Adaptive thermogenesis has been explored at length already on the Academy, but it will be touched on here then explored again in a later section for clarity.

Adaptive thermogenesis amounts to a reduction in TDEE that cannot be explained entirely by a lower bodyweight or reduction in NEAT (though the latter accounts for most of it). In order to potentially limit adaptation, but moreso in an effort to reduce the other negative effects of prolonged fat loss (such as hunger, lethargy, etc.) it is essential that regular diet breaks are considered. The precise protocol for doing this is outlined in the module on fat loss programming, but as a general overview and recap it is necessary to return calories to a maintenance level for a reasonable period of time (typically one week) periodically during a dieting phase. The frequency with which these breaks would occur rises with increasing leanness in an ideal world, and so a 24 week prep may take the following shape:

- Weeks 1-7: Lose 1.5% bodyweight per week

- Week 8: Maintain

- Weeks 9-15: Lose 1% bodyweight per week

- Week 16: Maintain

- Weeks 17-20: Lose 0.5% bodyweight per week

- Week 21: Maintain

- Weeks 22-24: Lose 0.25% bodyweight per week, on average

In those last three weeks it would be prudent, instead of being in a very small yet consistent deficit, to create the same deficit as the previous weeks (losing 0.5% of bodyweight) but to include regular refeeds every few days. A refeed is a single day (or even a few hours) where an individual eats a larger amount of food than they would during a diet. This is similar to a very short diet break and would hypothetically allow for slow fat loss to occur without any further short-term adaptive thermogenesis, at least according to the small amount of data pertaining to short-term crash dieting and refeeding (5). This is purely hypothetical, of course, but isn't without merit and must be considered in the context of broader and more concrete benefits.

As you have learned, circulating leptin decreases alongside reductions in bodyfat and this reduction acts to increase feeding behaviours through alterations in appetite signalling and food incentive salience and decreases in satiety signalling (6). Therefore, as individuals get exceptionally lean, it is to be expected that their serum leptin levels will decrease rapidly too. This results in much of the adaptations associated with extreme weight loss, such as significant and insatiable hunger, binge-eating tendencies and food fixation. This is then exacerbated because acute reductions in calorie intake (especially from carbohydrate) decrease leptin, because glucose is a necessary substrate for leptin production via the hexosamine biosynthetic pathway (6,7). As such the very act of dieting is likely to increase hunger exponentially, especially in the last few weeks of fat loss dieting. Because acute refeeds can counteract the acute reduction in leptin production associated with short-term caloric restriction in a very short space of time (5), it stands to reason that taking a 'diet for two days, refeed for one' approach in the last few weeks of competition preparation would make the final stretch far easier to adhere to. Seeing as this would minimise reductions in leptin and also remove longer stretches of calorie restriction, it could also be the case that this approach would mediate the muscle loss commonly associated with late-stage prep, generally categorised by an increase in dieting rapidity as noted earlier. This again, is purely hypothetical but worthy of consideration.

In an ideal situation, calorie restriction would end a few days prior to the show, allowing for the individual to increase their carbohydrate intake and replenish glycogen stores, as well as allowing them to get some much-needed sleep (which, as you will see, can be a problem for physique athletes). This will be fully explored when we discuss peaking.

As a final note, there is no real need during diet breaks to exceed calorie requirements and in fact doing so could be counterproductive, though it is important to raise them to maintenance, at least in the earlier stages of prep where doing so is possible. As noted in the MATADOR study (8), not doing so does not limit adaptive thermogenesis. The same typically applies to refeeds outside contexts we will discuss later.

The actual calorie deficit needed in order to achieve continuous fat loss will need to be continually monitored and adjusted. An athlete dieting on 2500kcals in the initial stages of prep may need to reduce this by 250 or more every few months, primarily due to being lighter and so having both a lower BMR and a reduced energy expenditure during activity (EAT and NEAT are reduced when you are lighter because locomotion requires less effort). This means that it is unlikely that the calorie target will be the same throughout a diet and should be considered to be dynamic. Perhaps the athlete starts with a 25% reduction in calories, and then another 10% reduction is applied to the current intake each time the client's weight remains stable for more than one week, meaning 2500kcals becomes 2250kcals, which then becomes 2000kcals, then 1800kcals and so on.

This will need to be monitored for the athlete in question, but 10% reductions over time are relatively commonplace, at least until the latter stages of prep where smaller adjustments may be needed. Importantly these should be done reactively rather than proactively – there is no need to reduce calories further when fat loss is occurring already. As a real-world example, one case study of a 67kg female competitor saw her drop from 2500kcals to just under 1500kcals over the space of 20 weeks (20).

In short, a calorie deficit must be sustained for the requisite time. Regular diet breaks are important in order to improve adherence, provide psychological breaks and potentially limit adaptive thermogenesis insofar as doing so is possible, and towards the latter stages these may need to be replaced by more acute phases of dieting and refeeding to increase adherence, mediate adaptation and potentially limit muscle loss. The prep should be allowed as much time as is needed, plus some additional time to account for plateaus, diet breaks, mistakes, holidays and miscalculations. If in doubt, add another few weeks. Now this has been explored, we can look at the next topic, macronutrients.

25.9. Macronutrient recommendations for contest prep

This section will look at the macronutrient recommendations for all but the last week of prep, which will be covered by the section on peaking. This is the section which is arguably the most straightforward, although it hasn't always been that way. Bodybuilding diets have been some of the most controversial within the fitness industry since time immemorial, and that is simply because bodybuilding is a sport that has thrived on anecdotal evidence for decades.

Before the dawn of the internet, research was extremely difficult and time consuming to come across. Those of us who have never lived without internet access can't really appreciate how much easier it is now that we have access to more or less any journal we want, simply by Googling. As little as three decades ago the only way to read research yourself was to go to university or look for it in paper library databases – suffice it to say a research paper that will take less than a minute to find now could have been well over a month away in the not too distant past. Therefore, the truth is that most bodybuilders just didn't have access to hard data. This then needs to be combined with the fact that, through virtue of being an extremely niche sport, bodybuilding literature has been historically thin on the ground. As a final barrier, natural bodybuilding is a very recent sport and so most direct bodybuilding research up until perhaps the early 2000's involved athletes using steroids. As such, bodybuilders were left with one option: ask the guys that are bigger than you what they did, and hopefully it'll work for you too. Gym culture was awash with local heroes who disseminated their opinions and findings to others and numerous 'done things' were born.

This anecdote-based practice has led to some very important realisations, garnered through trial and error by the athletes themselves. Even official advice pertaining to sports nutrition has focused heavily on carbohydrate intake for a long time, but bodybuilders adopted higher protein intakes very early on in the sport's rise to prominence. Similarly, bodybuilders realised relatively quickly that they could utilise regular high carbohydrate days during a dieting phase to reduce appetite and improve performance. However, this should not be taken as evidence that bodybuilders are 'ahead of the curve' because there are a number of really bad ideas that saw their inception in gyms, too. Eating extremely restrictive diets (stereotyped as chicken, broccoli and rice) with a very low-fat intake have been the norm for a long time, as have practices such as avoiding simple carbohydrates, avoiding carbohydrates altogether and also avoiding sodium.

Indeed the popularity of 'clean eating' and the idea that one cannot lose fat without it could arguably be traced back to the world of bodybuilding, as can the idea of eating 8-10 meals per day to 'stoke the metabolic fire'. Neither of these practices are something that should be advised, both because they are extremely difficult to adhere to and simply, they aren't necessary.

Fortunately there is more research available now, and much of it is relatively easy to locate and ready. Because of this, evidence-based nutritional practices by bodybuilders are becoming more common, with perhaps one area agreed upon by more than any other: the ideal macronutrient intake for competition prep.

The macronutrient intake for this aspect of the sport is somewhat different to the general advice that we have given so far because of the unique nature of bodybuilding prep. In order for a bodybuilder to get into the best shape possible they need to get exceptionally lean while also maintaining as much muscle mass as possible – something that is very difficult to do. Therefore, the first thing to look at is the macronutrient most likely to preserve muscle mass and the one of which bodybuilders had worked out the importance of, decades ago: protein.

In what could probably be considered the definitive work on the topic, Helms et al (9) note that research over the decades has repeatedly shown that roughly 2g of protein per kg/bw recommended to maximise hypertrophy (we recommend up to 2.2g per kilogram earlier in this course) is insufficient to avoid a negative nitrogen balance in a calorie deficit, even alongside exercise. The two figures that appear from reviews of the literature are 1.8-2.7g /kg/bw, as recommended by Phillips and Van Loon, and 2.3-3.1g per kilogram of lean body mass as per a different review by Helms et al (this review was considered within the broader review about which we are talking). It is likely that the second range is more likely to be appropriate for bodybuilders as it comes from a study looking at lean, resistance trained individuals in a calorie deficit, and so it is the figure we will stand by for the purpose of this module.

> **Note:** Lean body mass is calculated by subtracting bodyfat percentage from total body mass – so a 100kg individual at 20% bodyfat has 80kg of lean body mass.

This number needs to scale upwards with leanness and severity of the deficit. The exact manner in which you would enact this scaling is always going to be somewhat arbitrary until really specific recommendations can be made (and even then it's hard to make precise recommendations for individuals), but a reasonable way to plan it would be to opt for roughly 2.5g per kilogram of lean body mass until the athlete is 5% bodyfat above stage weight, then to go for roughly 3g per kilogram. Note that this is purely for illustration and you are free to come up with your own methods using trial and error, and/or according to athlete preference.

Next it is worth considering fat intake. We do this because calorie intake has already been set and so, by default, setting one of the other two macronutrients will simultaneously set the other, and consuming a diet that is too low in fat inhibits vitamin absorption as well as making dieting harder to do thanks to increased hunger. There is also some evidence that a diet too low in fat may hamper testosterone levels (9) though the literature is far from clear or conclusive on that front.

A recommendation of less than 35% has been recommended already in this course, and 20-30% is often recommended for athletes specifically (9) in the hopes that this will reduce the likelihood of negatively altering testosterone levels. The problem with this is caused by two interlinked factors:

- As already mentioned, increasing fat or carbohydrates within a given calorie allowance reduces carbohydrates or fats respectively, and this could represent a large chunk of someone's daily intake if they are already following our advice on protein, as above

- Decreasing carbohydrate too much can hamper training performance (9) and that could lead to increased muscle loss

As such it is prudent to set fat intake first, if only as a means of avoiding fat getting too low – but to what do we set it? As noted above 20-30% is theoretically a good intake for strength athletes to avoid hormonal decreases and maximise health, but unfortunately this is unrealistic for many. It's not unusual to see a 75kg natural bodybuilder dieting on as little as 1800kcal. Factoring in a protein intake of approximately 200g (800kcal) and 30% kcal from fat, totalling 600kcal, that leaves 400kcal or 100g of carbohydrate left over. To maximise performance, 4-7g of carbohydrate per kilogram of bodyweight is recommended – a bodybuilder will never be able to achieve this throughout prep but it's safe to say that in this example (where the total is 66% less than the minimum recommendation), performance will be hampered more than it needs to be. As such, a lower 15-20% fat diet is something that would be useful in this particular instance.

Carbohydrate would then simply make up the rest of allotted calories. A fibre recommendation is unlikely to be necessary because most bodybuilders will opt for high volume and low palatable foods (such as vegetables and fibrous starches) to reduce daily hunger, but nevertheless the recommendation of 10-15g per 1000kcal eaten, noted in an earlier module, will suffice.

To summarise, the nutritional approach during contest prep would look like the below for a 75kg individual at 15% bodyfat who is losing 1% bodyweight per week on 2200kcals:

- **Protein:** Lean body mass is 63kg, and as he has a little way to go protein doesn't need to be at the top end of the scale yet. He will opt for 2.5g per kilogram, so around 160g protein per day

- **Fat:** 20% of calories is 450kcal, or 50g of fat at 9kcal per gram

- **Carbohydrate:** This totals (160x4)+450=1090kcal. This leaves 1110kcal for carbohydrate, or just over 275g, including around 20-30g fibre

These macronutrients, much like is the case for building muscle mass, should be distributed primarily due to client preference. Most athletes will subjectively report feeling that they can train more effectively when placing carbohydrate around their workout, but this is not likely to be necessary for bodybuilders who only train once per day and so will have consumed a day's worth of carbohydrate at minimum in between training sessions (9). Protein distribution may be a little more important, because as noted in the module on hypertrophy, muscle protein synthesis is only elevated for a finite amount of time after each feeding. That said, the distribution of protein to maintain muscle is likely less important than that to gain it, so long as very low or very high intakes are avoided. Therefore, a recommendation of 3-6 protein feedings per day is appropriate.

As calories are reduced further throughout the diet to account for weight loss resulting in a reduced TDEE, it is likely that the reduction will come at the expense of carbohydrate because fat is set and, if anything, protein is likely to increase. This does unfortunately mean that the latter stages of contest prep will involve relatively low carbohydrate intakes by necessity, not because carbohydrates impede fat loss per se but because those calories have to come from somewhere. For example, the below would be the diet of the same individual at 8% bodyfat (for the sake of illustration assume he has lost 7% bodyfat and no muscle at all, though this is unlikely to be the case). He is now around 69kg, and his calories have reduced incrementally to be 1800kcal per day.

- **Protein:** Lean body mass is still around 63kg, but he is shooting for 3g per kilogram of lean body mass now so his protein intake will be around 190g per day

- **Fat:** 20% of calories is now 360, meaning 40g fat

- **Carbohydrate:** This totals (190x4)+360=1120kcal. This only leaves 680kcal for carbohydrate, or just over 170g of carbohydrate, including around 20-30g fibre

This is going to leave the athlete hungry and depleted, potentially risking poor adherence and certainly risking a drop in exercise performance – an independent risk factor for muscle loss. This is one reason why regular refeeds become important during the last few weeks of competition prep. These would probably be included once every 1-2 weeks (as well as diet breaks) when the client starts to subjectively feel that training performance is being hampered by the severity of the diet. It is difficult to provide more specific advice for this because the particulars of the training volume and frequency will play a major role in the timing of acute refeeds. Regardless of this, the approach would be the same – increase carbohydrate until the client is roughly at a maintenance calorie intake for one day. Looking at the dietary setup above (listed again below) this would likely start to be introduced around week 10 or so with a refeed every two weeks. At week 15 this might be increased to weekly refeeds, then as mentioned already at week 21 the refeeds would occur every 3-4 days.

- Weeks 1-7: Lose 1.5% bodyweight per week

- Week 8: Maintain

- Weeks 9-15: Lose 1% bodyweight per week

- Week 16: Maintain

- Weeks 17-20: Lose 0.5% bodyweight per week

- Week 21: Maintain

- Weeks 22-24: Lose 0.25% bodyweight per week, on average

Note: These refeeds would not be calculated into the client's weekly average until the last couple of weeks. If the client needs 2800kcal to maintain and is eating roughly 2250kcal for a 20% deficit, they would eat this each day alongside one day at 2800kcal that focused primarily on carbohydrate intake to refill glycogen stores and potentially increase leptin for a very short time. This should not inhibit fat loss across the week, though it will inhibit it on that specific day, meaning you will need to ensure the client buys in to the idea. Many athletes worry so much about losing fat that the idea of not losing it for one day every two weeks is unattractive. Helping them understand that maintaining training performance and therefore muscle mass, should go some way towards convincing them of the benefits. As always, we must respect the client's wishes and autonomy but helping them see how this approach aligns with their values and needs lets them make a truly informed decision.

As a final note on this section, it is worth considering food choice. Like at any other time of the year there should be no banned foods or things that are off limits, but that does come with a substantial caveat. During times of energy restriction an athlete will be hungry, and this will be exacerbated as the client gets leaner for reasons of which you are already aware (reread the module on programming fat loss for a refresher). This means that food choices will need to be primarily whole foods, focusing on protein, fibre and overall food volume most of the time. Cravings should not be ignored and there is no need to adopt a clean eating approach, but at the same time a cost:benefit analysis will need to be performed for athletes looking to utilise 50% of their daily calorie intake for a burger. This is where refeeds and diet breaks can come in handy, because they allow for increased calorie intake and thus, flexibility.

25.10. Peak week nutrition

The above approach is relatively simple: consume a calorie deficit while focusing primarily on ensuring adequate protein and carbohydrate, for enough time that you end up extremely lean. Within that, diet breaks and refeeds may help with reducing muscle loss as well as hunger, and gradual decreases in caloric intake will need to be utilised over time to ensure fat loss keeps happening.

What is not so simple is the nutritional approach needed for the last week or so before the competition, known as peak week. During peak week the goal is not to lose fat – fat loss should already be achieved by this point. Instead the purpose is to manipulate certain variables (primarily water stores within the body) to ensure you look as big and 'full' as possible on stage. The golden rule here, however, is to avoid making your client look 50% worse in order to try to get 5% better. If in doubt, ignore peak week entirely.

Three approaches typically utilised in this period are sodium, water and carbohydrate manipulation. It is usually the case that around one week from show day, the athlete will start to decrease sodium intake incrementally, as well as decreasing water intake from around three days out. The idea here is to reduce as much water retention as possible and 'dry out'. Athletes will also generally increase training volume until around three days out to deplete glycogen, followed by an increase in carbohydrate intake to refill glycogen stores – a similar approach to that often adopted by carbohydrate loading endurance athletes. The idea is to reduce subcutaneous water, and simultaneously increase glycogen and glycogen-associated water storage within muscle tissue.

Below is a table that highlights what actually happens over a six day period of sodium depletion (10):

Fig. 76

	Baseline	Day 1	Day 2	Day 6
Urinary sodium	217 (mmol/day)	105	59	9.9
Aldosterone	10.4 (ng/100ml)	11.7	22.5	37
Serum sodium	139 (mEq/L)	139	139	138

What you see is that the participants' bodies fought to keep serum sodium even. They did this by increasing aldosterone, the hormone responsible for causing reabsorption of sodium from the kidneys rather than excretion in urine, and so preventing sodium being removed. Unfortunately, along with an increase in sodium reabsorption in the kidneys, a reabsorption of water occurs too, thanks to the osmotic pressure created. Put simply, the kidneys reabsorb sodium into the local blood supply from the urine, and that increases the concentration of sodium in the local blood. That effectively results in water being 'sucked' out too and the final outcome is that serum (blood) sodium stays roughly the same, and some of that additional water winds up in the extracellular compartment, leading to water retention: the very thing the bodybuilder was trying to avoid!

Sodium manipulation is a bad idea. Along with being ineffective, it can cause a number of health problems ranging from cramp (11) to death (12), and so it should be avoided. Cutting water has obvious health consequences but what may be less obvious are the physique related issues – put simply you cannot realistically control where water is lost from when you become voluntarily dehydrated and so it is wishful thinking to believe that water will be lost from subcutaneous tissue only, sparing muscular water.

Human muscle is roughly 70% water when you are properly hydrated (13), and during dehydration it is unlikely that the relative amounts of intracellular and extracellular water will shift in the manner you want. In fact, because extracellular water (water under your skin, in your lymphatic system and in your blood) is more important in the short-term, during dehydration intracellular water is sacrificed to maintain it (14). This means that dehydration will make your muscles look flat, rather than making you look 'dry'. Much like sodium manipulation, water manipulation should be ignored.

The only possible exception to this would be a small reduction in water the day of the show in order to reduce stomach distention. Drink only to thirst and sip water prior to going on stage – beyond that, stay hydrated. As for your sodium intake, maintaining your usual salt intake year-round is a perfectly good strategy. The only exception is for a female client who is about to menstruate and so who is likely to gain water. If this is the case, dropping sodium in the day before/of the show could be an effective strategy.

The final approach in peak week, carbohydrate loading, potentially has more efficacy. As the client has been in a significant calorie deficit (albeit one that is punctuated by refeeds), they are likely to store far less glycogen than they otherwise would. It is well known in bodybuilding circles that you look bigger the day after a carbohydrate refeed, and many report looking leaner (likely because 'fuller' muscles are pressing against their skin more effectively). Indeed, in one study participants who used carbohydrate loading had a biceps that measured 4.9% larger than it did six weeks prior (9), a result unlikely to be down to actual muscular hypertrophy during a depleted period. The method of working out a carbohydrate load is through trial and error, ideally using the last two weeks of prep to do it and adhering to carbohydrate intakes seen as carbohydrate loading in endurance athletes. The final two weeks may look like this:

- **14 days out:** Refeed by increasing carbohydrate to 7g per kilogram of bodyweight (the amount suggested as being adequate for strength athletes), and slightly decreasing protein and fat to 2g per kilogram and 15% of dieting intake, respectively

- **13 days out:** Assess physique, eat dieting calories

- **12 days out:** Assess physique, eat dieting calories

- **11 days out:** Assess physique, eat dieting calories

- **10 days out:** Assess physique, eat dieting calories

- **9 days out:** Did the client look full, or did you need more carbohydrate? If so, try 8g per kilogram. If not, refeed as usual by increasing to maintenance

- **8-4 days out:** Assess physique. Which day did the client look best? The day after the refeed or the day after that? And which time, the higher or lower intake amount? Whichever worked best, you now know the approach you need for the next 3 days

- **3 days out:** Eat at maintenance or refeed if client looked better after 3 days

- **2 days out:** Eat at maintenance or refeed if client looked better after 2 days

- **1 day out:** Refeed, or eat at maintenance if already done

The only other important factor would be to ensure fibre intake was relatively low the day before/day of the show. The last thing you need is a fibre-distended stomach! Focusing on easy to digest foods like fish and white rice will be hugely helpful, as will sugary foods like sweet cereal.

This approach may not appear as glamorous and exciting as the idea of altering sodium and water, but truthfully that doesn't matter. As already said, the first goal of peaking should be to avoid making the client look 50% worse in order to try to look 5% better! An alternative strategy for peak week would be to refeed with roughly 150% of your usual refeed carbohydrates on Monday (shows are almost always on Saturday), then eat at maintenance during the week. You could then consume your usual refeed carbohydrate intake on Thursday and assess what you need to do on Friday – be that a few press-ups and bodyweight squats to deplete excess carbohydrate 'spill over', or another carbohydrate load, depending on whether you look like you've gained water, or whether you're looking flat.

25.11. Training during prep

During peak week, the training you do is similarly important, as indeed it is in the rest of prep. During prep itself there is no consensus on how to manipulate training variables. Many trainees change training significantly, often decreasing training intensity (weight lifted) and increasing volume and frequency. The idea here stems from the fact that an increase in volume is critical for muscle growth (16) and so keeping it high makes sense for this reason, as well as because higher volume training logically burns more calories, and of course it's easier to squat lighter when you're feeling fatigued. This may be mistaken, though.

During the initial stages of a diet an athlete should be able to train more or less as normal – they are relatively well fuelled and should still be able to make progress as they always would, perhaps resulting in some recomposition. As fatigue starts to set in, however, the athlete must choose between reducing volume or reducing intensity because both cannot be maintained – evidence seems to suggest that maintaining intensity is the most important factor rather than volume. In fact, in one interesting study on the topic, participants trained for 16 weeks then detrained using either 1/3 or 1/9 of the volume, or they stopped completely. The group using 1/9 the volume didn't lose any muscle, while the group using 1/3 of the volume also maintained some muscle fibre adaptations that helped improve strength outside of hypertrophy (17). This suggests that a trainee would be better to drop to 2-3 sets with a heavy weight, rather than keeping 4 sets, increasing the volume and reducing the load. Of course, at some point it may be the case that load does need to reduce, too, but this should be avoided as much as possible – tension overload is the primary driver for muscle protein synthesis (16), and during a diet when MPS is lower than it otherwise would be, keeping it as high as possible should be the aim. This attempt to maintain and even build strength (successfully or not) throughout prep should continue until the final week.

Training has historically been cut during the final week in an effort to maintain glycogen stores, but this is potentially a mistake, because resistance training increases muscle glucose uptake independently of, and due to, an increase in insulin sensitivity (GLUT4 is translocated without insulin, and insulin-mediated translocation is increased, too) (15). As such it is wise not to stop training, potentially until the Friday, as this could help to increase muscular update of the final carbohydrate load.

As this is the final week it is unlikely that muscle retention will be an issue and therefore more 'pump' training could be done in order to help the client reduce allostatic load and increase glucose uptake. A reduction in allostatic load (which could be high by this point in prep thanks to the stress of being hungry and tired) may help to reduce the amount of aldosterone receptor binding and activation by cortisol, and so could reduce water retention leading up to show day.

As a last point, cardiovascular training is really common for bodybuilding preparation as a means of increasing calorie expenditure, but this like all tools should be used sparingly and only when needed. The ideal prep would involve no cardio and so coaches and athletes should start there, adding it in when weight loss stalls or when the athlete/client would prefer doing that (and can recover from it) to food restriction. Both tools are important and both will ultimately be used by almost all competitors. However, just like it wouldn't be good practice to adopt a 50% deficit out of the gate for prep, adding in 5 cardio sessions per week at week 1 is unwise. Adding in 30 minute blocks as you go, as necessary, is sufficient and it could be argued that walking or other low impact forms of cardio are preferable as these do not impinge upon recovery, allowing for a greater focus on gym work.

With all of that covered, it is pertinent for us to discuss the darker side of bodybuilding prep. After all looking to achieve extreme levels of leanness is not likely to result in a healthy outcome.

25.12. Health consequences of prep

While it falls under the umbrella of fitness, this is really a misnomer when it comes to bodybuilding prep because a bodybuilder in prep would be considered anything other than the typical definition of the term. Bodybuilders during prep are tired, they feel weak and typically struggle sleeping, with one paper reporting that bodybuilders become more fatigued, depressed, tense, confused, and less vigorous over time (22), and it shouldn't surprise you to learn that this reflects changes occurring on a biological level.

First of all, we need to consider the significant risk of muscle loss. You learned about this extensively in the module on programming nutrition for fat loss, so we will not explore it in great detail here. Suffice it to say that bodybuilding prep is the situation representing more risk of muscle loss than any other in fitness because it involves large reductions in calories with very lean people. Ensuring protein intake and resistance training are on point is critical for success and should be considered the second most important thing after a calorie deficit for this period.

Energy restriction decreases sympathetic nervous system output (18), and of course alongside this leptin will be reduced significantly due to energy restriction and fat loss per se, as you learned in the module on programming fat loss. What this means is that prep will be associated with increased fatigue and hunger. General feelings of tiredness and a lack of motivation are extremely common in our experience, but this is not the only psychological issue at hand.

Bodybuilders during prep are prone to binge eating and other eating disorders, body dysmorphia, anger, short temper and anxiety (9) and so undergoing the process while any of these issues are already present or historically have been an issue must be considered very carefully. The decreased sympathetic nervous tone will also come with a reduction in day to day muscle tone, including facially, leading to 'prep face' – while low energy intake and fatigue impairs cognition resulting in 'prep brain' and slurred words.

Bodybuilding prep can also cause havoc hormonally for both sexes. One female athlete tracked during a moderate prep including sensible calorie restriction and moderate amounts of cardiovascular exercise followed by a proper period of recovery, experienced menstrual disruption in month one of prep and lost her cycle at week 10 of 20. It did not recover until 71 weeks post-show despite a return to a healthy weight and food intake within 20 weeks (19). A male competitor followed as a case study showed similar issues, with the below graph indicating the changes in his hormonal secretion during the course of the study (21):

Fig. 77

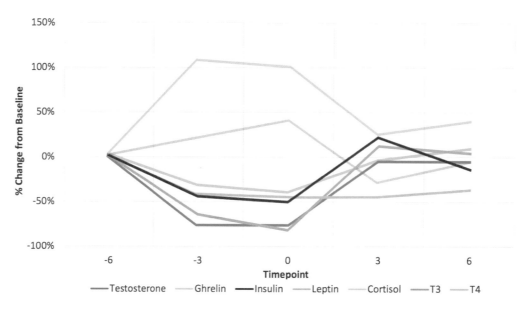

As you can see, testosterone, insulin, leptin, and thyroid hormone levels all dipped pretty extremely, while grehlin and cortisol both skyrocketed. This is likely to reflect an extreme lack of energy and drive, a lot of hunger and a lack of sexual function that did not recover until 6 months after the study. Leptin didn't return at all, though this could be because he was still lighter than he was at baseline after 6 months of recovery.

The increase in cortisol is likely to coincide with a decrease in immune function and the associated increase in susceptibility to infections and illnesses, while the decreased thyroid function can make the individual feel cold and weak. The thing to remember here is that both of these competitors underwent relatively well planned and executed approaches and so had theoretically done all that was possible in order to reduce risk and come out of prep in the healthiest way possible. While we can minimise the damage, we cannot eradicate it, and so anyone looking to get to extreme levels of leanness should be made aware that the practice comes with some risks, and with some inevitabilities – a loss of menstrual cycle and large dip in testosterone being two of these.

25.13. Post-show nutrition and rebounding

Finally, we need to look at the last piece of the puzzle, what to do after the show. In recent years a discussion around 'reverse dieting' has been at the foreground. This approach involves slow incremental increases in calorie intake after the show, in an effort to reduce fat gain. The basic assumption is that adaptive thermogenesis will mean the client has a lower TDEE than would be anticipated and so an increase of calories which matches a calculated TDEE would cause the client to rebound and gain weight. Indeed, as we're sure you know, most people who lose weight do end up regaining it over time. One study in clinical obese patients found that as little as 5% of people maintained weight loss after as little as 6 years (23).

The problem here is that this study involves clinically obese people, for whom weight regain is a problem. However as you have just seen, achieving the level of leanness needed for bodybuilding is not healthy at all, and in fact regain is accompanied by a return to greater general health. What this means is that regain is not undesirable, and in fact a bodybuilder would do well to try to gain a small amount of bodyfat as fast as possible after the show until they reach a healthy bodyfat level (which will still be extremely lean by most standards). This is another reason why bodybuilding should not be undertaken by those with pronounced body dysmorphia or other eating disorder tendencies.

The remainder of the argument hinges on the idea that the athlete's metabolic rate will be severely reduced and so increasing calories a lot straight away results in a large surplus, but this isn't true. Remember, even after extremely rapid and arguably reckless fat loss, adaptation only accounted for around a 14% reduction in BMR (24). This means that even if you did want to eliminate fat loss, you could still jump to your predicted TDEE, minus roughly 15% of your BMR, and that's assuming you have adaptation equivalent to the worst recorded cases in the literature.

In fact, the approach taken by the male participant in the case study mentioned earlier is the approach that most athletes would do well to take, as illustrated below (21):

Fig. 78

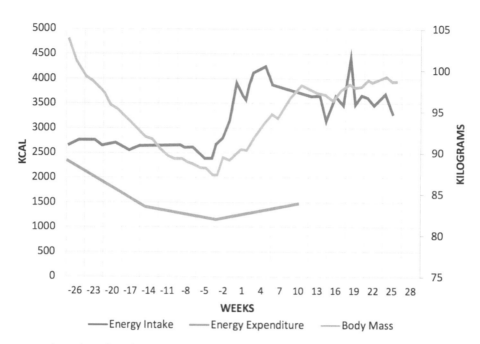

Here you see that his food intake dramatically and rapidly increased after the show, accompanied by a return to close to baseline of his bodyweight. If you compare this to the earlier graph of his hormone levels you will see that the rate of endocrine recovery tracks very closely on to the recovery of bodyweight, indicating the importance of doing this. You also see that his energy expenditure (this is RMR) decreased over the course of the study, then began to increase again alongside weight and his energy intake. Unfortunately his EE is not measured beyond 13 weeks but it's not unreasonable to assume that this would recover alongside everything else, it would perhaps be a little lower as his weight (and thus leptin) did not return to baseline.

Similarly, the female client from earlier (19) brought her calories back to the same level that they were at the start of prep within two weeks of the show, before gradually increasing them to create an energy surplus for the off-season, as illustrated below:

Fig. 79

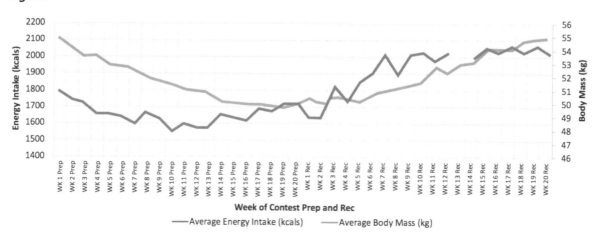

Increasing calories slowly post-show is a bad idea, because typically an athlete will be in a significant calorie deficit at that point, and so adding small amounts of calories will not put them in a surplus (and so won't allow them to regain healthy weight) but will instead reduce the size of the deficit and keep the client dieting for a longer period than is necessary – possibly exacerbating all of the aforementioned psychophysiological issues. To give a more formulaic approach to post-show recovery, the following method is a good one:

- **Show day:** In the evening the client can eat whatever they desire but should not binge. Binge eating post-show is extremely common and could result in a problematic behaviour cycle. If this is not likely to be possible, consider tracking calories at this time and aiming to hit their refeed targets

- **Day 1 post-show:** Calculate estimated TDEE, then subtract 15% of BMR from this figure. Do not panic when weight gain is seen on the scales as they will likely increase glycogen stores and gain weight via undigested food (remember, they've eaten low fibre for two days!)

- **Day 4 post-show:** Increase to calculated TDEE

- **Day 7 post-show:** Increase to small surplus

You will almost certainly find that their calories need to go a lot higher than they are at day 7 in order to gain weight. As they eat more, leptin and thyroid hormones will recover and sympathetic nervous tone will increase, and all of this will lead to improved NEAT, reduced mitochondrial efficiency and increased ability to train hard. This in turn will increase TDEE and will need to be accounted for. Adding an additional 5% of calorie intake per week until scale weight increases is a good approach, followed by monitoring and increasing again over time.

As a final consideration, it would not be a bad idea to have private blood testing done before prep, a day or two after the show, and then again every 12 weeks or so. This will help the client monitor their hormone levels and know when you have recovered fully from the experience.

25.14. Summary

In many ways bodybuilding contest preparation is like a typical fat loss diet. A calorie surplus is applied alongside a moderate to high protein intake and resistance training to retain muscle mass, and then calorie intake and cardio is adjusted over time to ensure fat loss persists. At the same time some other considerations become very important, including management of hunger, resistance training intensity and moderate amounts of cardiovascular training. Provided enough time is allotted to reach show condition and the athlete is able to adhere to the diet, they should have no problem reaching the best condition they could achieve, though as you have learned throughout this course, a tough diet will necessitate a lot of support from both the coach and the rest of the client's immediate circle.

Arguably the psychological side of prep Is the hardest. A client will need support in terms of motivation (which should come internally, through recognition of values and a mindset of approaching a challenge rather than suffering an ordeal), and in terms of self-confidence.

Most people overestimate muscle mass and underestimate fat mass, and so the athlete expecting to be shredded at 80kg may be disheartened when they see themselves at 75kg with a long way to go. This is where the coach needs to step in to reassure and to provide objective analysis. Regular photographs, perhaps biweekly down to weekly depending on the distance from show day, are an incredibly useful tool for showing the client that they are making progress and not just getting smaller.

Ultimately bodybuilding prep and the derivatives thereof is a massive yet rewarding challenge for those who decide to undertake it willingly and with enthusiasm, but it isn't for everyone and a judgement call will need to be made. A client who decides 8 weeks out that this isn't for them because they hate feeling tired and their lack of a sex drive is harming their relationship should be encouraged to do what it is they really value (at the same time someone wanting to quit two weeks out because they feel small in clothes while looking great during posing practice may just need a pat on the back).

Whatever the reason for doing it, the focus during bodybuilding prep should be maximal muscle retention and maximal fat loss, but the priorities need to change afterwards. Post-show the athlete needs to focus on getting healthy as quickly as possible, and that is likely to involve gaining 5% bodyfat or so. Preparing for this long before show day will be critical because being in amazing shape by bodybuilding standards can be addictive for some. A responsible coach never shirks this responsibility, and so it goes almost without saying that your goal is not just to get a client lean.

The goal of a prep coach is to get the client lean in the healthiest way possible, and then get them back to normality. Leaving clients after a show is a potential recipe for disaster.

25.15. References

1. Andersen, R., Barlett, S., Morgan, G. and Brownell, K. (1995). Weight loss, psychological, and nutritional patterns in competitive male body builders. International Journal of Eating Disorders, 18(1), pp.49-57.

2. Forbes, G. (2006). Body Fat Content Influences the Body Composition Response to Nutrition and Exercise. Annals of the New York Academy of Sciences, 904(1), pp.359-365.

3. Heymsfield, S., Gonzalez, M., Shen, W., Redman, L. and Thomas, D. (2014). Weight loss composition is one-fourth fat-free mass: a critical review and critique of this widely cited rule. Obesity Reviews, 15(4), pp.310-321.

4. Newton, L., Hunter, G., Bammon, M. and Roney, R. (1993). Changes in Psychological State and Self-Reported Diet During Various Phases of Training in Competitive Bodybuilders. Journal of Strength and Conditioning Research, 7(3), pp.153-158.

5. Monteleone, P., Bortolotti, F., Fabrazzo, M., La Rocca, A., Fuschino, A. and Maj, M. (2000). Plasma Leptin Response to Acute Fasting and Refeeding in Untreated Women with Bulimia Nervosa. The Journal of Clinical Endocrinology & Metabolism, 85(7), pp.2499-2503.

6. Farr, O., Gavrieli, A. and Mantzoros, C. (2015). Leptin applications in 2015. Current Opinion in Endocrinology & Diabetes and Obesity, 22(5), pp.353-359.

7. Considine, R., Cooksey, R., Williams, L., Fawcett, R., Zhang, P., Ambrosius, W., Whitfield, R., Jones, R., Inman, M., Huse, J. and McClain, D. (2000). Hexosamines Regulate Leptin Production in Human Subcutaneous Adipocytes1. The Journal of Clinical Endocrinology & Metabolism, 85(10), pp.3551-3556.

8. Byrne, N., Sainsbury, A., King, N., Hills, A. and Wood, R. (2017). Intermittent energy restriction improves weight loss efficiency in obese men: the MATADOR study. International Journal of Obesity, 42(2), pp.129-138.

9. Helms, E., Aragon, A. and Fitschen, P. (2014). Evidence-based recommendations for natural bodybuilding contest preparation: nutrition and supplementation. Journal of the International Society of Sports Nutrition, 11(1), p.20.

10. Rogacz, S., Williams, G. and Hollenberg, N. (1990). Time course of enhanced adrenal responsiveness to angiotensin on a low salt diet. Hypertension, 15(4), pp.376-380.

11. Young, G. (2009). Leg Cramps. BMJ Clinical Evidence, 2009(1113).

12. Mohan, S., Gu, S., Parikh, A. and Radhakrishnan, J. (2013). Prevalence of Hyponatremia and Association with Mortality: Results from NHANES. The American Journal of Medicine, 126(12), pp.1127-1137.e1.

13. Institute of Medicine of the National Academies. Water. Dietary Reference Intakes for Water, Sodium, Chloride, Potassium and Sulfate. Washington, D.C: National Academy Press; 2005. pp. 73–185.

14. Nose, H., Mack, G., Shi, X. and Nadel, E. (1988). Shift in body fluid compartments after dehydration in humans. Journal of Applied Physiology, 65(1), pp.318-324.

15. Richter, E. and Hargreaves, M. (2013). Exercise, GLUT4, and Skeletal Muscle Glucose Uptake. Physiological Reviews, 93(3), pp.993-1017.

16. Schoenfeld, B. (2010). The Mechanisms of Muscle Hypertrophy and Their Application to Resistance Training. Journal of Strength and Conditioning Research, 24(10), pp.2857-2872.

17. Bickel, C., Cross, J. and Bamman, M. (2011). Exercise Dosing to Retain Resistance Training Adaptations in Young and Older Adults. Medicine & Science in Sports & Exercise, 43(7), pp.1177-1187.

18. De Jonge, L., Moreira, E., Martin, C. and Ravussin, E. (2009). Impact of 6-month Caloric Restriction on Autonomic Nervous System Activity in Healthy, Overweight, Individuals. Obesity, 18(2), pp.414-416.

19. Halliday, T., Loenneke, J. and Davy, B. (2016). Dietary Intake, Body Composition, and Menstrual Cycle Changes during Competition Preparation and Recovery in a Drug-Free Figure Competitor: A Case Study. Nutrients, 8(11), p.740.

20. Rohrig, B. J., Pettitt, R. W., Pettitt, C. D., & Kanzenbach, T. L. (2017). Psycho-physiological Tracking of a Female Physique Competitor through Competition Preparation. International Journal of Exercise Science, 10(2), 301–311.

21. Rossow, L., Fukuda, D., Fahs, C., Loenneke, J. and Stout, J. (2013). Natural Bodybuilding Competition Preparation and Recovery: A 12-Month Case Study. International Journal of Sports Physiology and Performance, 8(5), pp.582-592.

22. Newton, L., Hunter, G., Bammon, M. and Roney, R. (1993). Changes in Psychological State and Self-Reported Diet During Various Phases of Training in Competitive Bodybuilders. Journal of Strength and Conditioning Research, 7(3), pp.153-158.

23. Grattan, B. and Connolly-Schoonen, J. (2012). Addressing Weight Loss Recidivism: A Clinical Focus on Metabolic Rate and the Psychological Aspects of Obesity. ISRN Obesity, 2012, pp.1-5.

24. Knuth, N., Johannsen, D., Tamboli, R., Marks-Shulman, P., Huizenga, R., Chen, K., Abumrad, N., Ravussin, E. and Hall, K. (2014). Metabolic adaptation following massive weight loss is related to the degree of energy imbalance and changes in circulating leptin. Obesity, p.n/a-n/a.

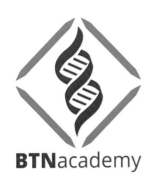

MODULE 26

NUTRITIONAL CONSIDERATIONS FOR MAKING WEIGHT

BTNacademy

26. MODULE 26: NUTRITIONAL CONSIDERATIONS FOR MAKING WEIGHT

26.1. Module aims

- To explain what making weight means, and outline the weight categories for boxing, kickboxing, MMA, powerlifting and Olympic lifting

- To inform students about weigh-ins and the timing thereof

- To give ideas around how to choose a weight class properly

- To provide the ideal scenario – how do you make weight in the healthiest and safest way possible?

- To advise around when the above cannot happen due to a lack of time

26.2. Key principles from module 25

In the last module we covered the process of prep for bodybuilding or similar endeavours – the process of getting extremely, unsustainably lean for competition. You learned:

- There are better and worse reasons for competing and understanding a client's why is critical before setting out. There may be some clients that should not consider prep and it would not be ethical for you to abstain from discussing this with them

- The level of leanness and muscularity is specific to the sport, so always be aware of the particular one you're looking to work in

- Physiques should always be judged without a pump, in bad lighting

- The duration of the prep should be roughly twice the percentage points of bodyfat a client would like to lose. Plan 16 weeks to lose 8%, for example. If in doubt go longer, but all fat should be lost by one week out

- Aim for 0.5-1.5% bodyweight loss per week

- Macronutrients would ideally include 2.3-3.1g of protein per kilogram of bodyweight, enough fat to cover absolute need and as much carbohydrate as remaining calorie needs will allow

- Lose fast at the start, and slower towards the end

- Diet breaks and refeeds will be important, especially as competition day approaches

- In peak week the golden rule is not to look worse in an effort to look better. Minimal changes should be done. Roughly two weeks out attempt a carbohydrate load, then use what you learn there to plan the 'real' one

- After the competition, get into a small surplus as fast as possible

- Negative endocrine effects are larely unavoidable, though recovery is possible provided proper eating resumes as quickly as possible. Do not attempt another prep before recovery has completely occurred, unless you really have to. Hormone testing before and after prep is a good idea

26.3.   Introduction to nutritional considerations for making weight

Making weight both safely and ethically for a fighter or lifter takes precision and a thorough understanding of the weight categories themselves, the nutritional requirements of the sport in question (and competition preparation) and a good understanding of refuelling strategies. Weight classes are used in a number of sports to differentiate between competitors in order to make competitions somewhat even. For example, pitting a 130kg fighter against a 47kg fighter would be unfair, and the same goes for strength and power sports too, but due to differing heights and genetic structures, as well as personal preferences, both kinds of athlete exist and wish to compete. Weight classes are typically ranges within which a competitor needs to be, for example a powerlifter competing in the 90kg class needs to be less than 90kg, but heavier than 83kg which is the upper limit of the class below. However, most of the time athletes do not walk around at their competition weight.

Carrying a little more weight than they compete with allows an athlete to fuel their training more effectively and potentially improve more between events, but this inevitably means losing weight ahead of a competition. This presents a number of challenges and nuanced approaches depending on some of the specific circumstances relevant to the situation, and so this is the topic of the present module.

26.4.   What are the weight classes?

As mentioned, the first thing to do is to become accustomed to the idea of weight classes and understand what they are (1). The classes athletes compete in differ between sports and even within a given sport they may differ between federations. It is because of this that the below should be seen as an example, and you should consult the rules of the particular sport for which you are hoping to prepare an athlete, in order to find out the boundaries to which you need to adhere.

The first thing to note is that the lower limit of a weight class is equal to the upper weight limit of the class below it, so as mentioned the 90kg powerlifting class ends at that weight and begins at 83kg which is the upper limit of the class below. We will state up front that realistically the vast majority of competitors stay rather close to the top end of their weight class because when all else is equal, a larger athlete is a stronger and more powerful one. A lean and well trained 75kg athlete has a large advantage over a lean and well trained 68kg athlete though they both fit in the same class for some sports.

Rules vary regarding competing outside of your weight class. Although professional fighters in many sports may fight above their weight class if they choose, an amateur fighter's weight must not fall below the lower limit. Some strength sports will allow you to move up a weight class but some will not, and there is also a variance for both sports regarding the rules surrounding missing weight, meaning weighing in too heavy. If an athlete is hoping to compete at 75kg but weighs in at 77kg on the day, they may be penalised in terms of points or score, they may not be able to compete, or they may have to compete in the higher weight category where, arguably, they will be at a significant disadvantage. Some example weight classes are listed below.

In Olympic lifting, athletes compete in a division determined by their body mass. There have been eight male divisions and eight female divisions since 2017 (2):

Fig. 80

Men	Women
56kg	48kg
62kg	53kg
69kg	58kg
77kg	63kg
85kg	69kg
94kg	75kg
105kg	90kg
105kg+	90kg+

Most powerlifting federations use the following weight classes:

Fig. 81

Men	Women
52kg	44kg
56kg	48kg
60kg	52kg
67.5kg	56kg
75kg	60kg
83kg	67.5kg
90kg	75kg
100kg	82.5kg
110kg	90kg
125kg	90kg+
140kg	
140kg+	

However, in 2011, the IPF (a drug tested organisation) introduced the following new weight classes (see overleaf):

Fig. 82

Men	Women
Up to 53kg (sub junior/junior)	43kg (sub junior/junior)
59kg	47kg
66kg	52kg
74kg	57kg
83kg	63kg
93kg	72kg
105kg	84kg
120kg	84kg+
120kg+	

In the UFC, like most fight sports, there is a name for each class. Men and women compete in the same weight classes, though often female competitors only compete in the lower end classes. Atomweight was added almost specifically for female athletes.

Fig. 83

Weight class	Upper limit
Atomweight	105lbs (48 kg)
Strawweight	115lbs (52.2 kg)
Flyweight	125lbs (56.7 kg)
Bantamweight	135lbs (61.2 kg)
Featherweight	145lbs (65.8 kg)
Lightweight	155lbs (70.3 kg)
Welterweight	170lbs (77.1 kg)
Middleweight	185lbs (83.9 kg)
Light heavyweight	205lbs (93.0 kg)
Heavyweight	265lbs (120.2 kg)

These examples should illustrate the vast array of weight classes seen in various different sports and give you some idea of the magnitude of difference between them. Generally weight classes move up in roughly 5-7kg jumps until around 90kg, at which point the bands get larger. As noted, it's necessary to find out the specific classes relevant to the competition you're looking at, at the time.

26.5.   What is making weight?

Making weight is term used by all fighting federations and competitive weight category sports. As we've discussed briefly already, hitting somewhere between an upper and lower target weight is important to allow a fair competition in both fight sports and lifting sports. We have also already mentioned that most competitors walk around heavier than their competition weight. This is typically because it allows for more fuel for training and so an athlete will gain weight in between competitions, but at the same time a new athlete (or even some experienced ones) may choose to compete in a lower category than their current bodyweight and so must lose weight to 'drop down a class' before the competition. There are numerous reasons for this, some of which are listed below:

- The weight class in which you compete is typically dictated by lean body mass, which as you know is slow to increase. This means that an athlete who walks around at 70kg must either:

  - Compete at 70kg in the 75kg class. This means they will be 5kg smaller than most other competitors and so at a disadvantage

  - Gain 5kg to reach the top of the class with everyone else, sacrificing body composition in the process and so generally, finding themselves far slower due to excess body fat

  - Lose weight to reach the upper limit of the lower 67.5kg class, which is far easier and likely to be more effective

- In strength sports the difference in lifts between weight classes can be quite large. Someone may find that their strength is competitive at a lower class but not at a higher one, so they will be tempted to drop weight in order to win despite this actually costing them a little in terms of their own personal lifting records. For example an athlete may squat 300kg at 90kg and come 3rd, but if they can drop to 83kg and squat 280kg they may break federation records

- As you will see later, many athletes opt to cut weight using water and glycogen manipulation, then regain that weight before the contest and so gain a significant weight advantage. This is possible when a weigh in is a long time before the competition, often it is 24 hours, and so could be considered part of the sport. Some famous MMA fighters, for example, will weigh in and meet weight then go home and come back the following day 5kg or more heavier (this is well within the rules). However, there are downsides to this approach, and if refuelling is not done properly a dehydrated and depleted athlete is at a huge disadvantage

Making weight has been referred to as the single most difficult aspect of partaking in a weight category sport, but as mentioned above cutting weight is a skill unto itself, that is large part of the job for professional athletes on a regular basis. Athletes who agree to compete in a specific weight class are expected to show up and make weight, and if they don't they are typically penalised or disqualified outright. As such there are two things done by fighters to make sure they are at the correct weight to compete, namely:

- Losing weight

- Cutting weight

These are different and require separate approaches. Losing weight (fat) is something that we have already discussed at length on this course and so we won't go much further into it here. Cutting weight, on the other hand, means short-term manipulation of bodyweight in the days before a competition, with the intention of refeeding and regaining this weight immediately (or in as short a space of time as possible) after being weighed. Cutting is typically done by manipulating glycogen and body water. This means that athletes need to balance the risk and reward of using large weight cuts and managing to refeed (so competing heavier, but risking being depleted), and using smaller cuts, or indeed not doing it at all, and coming in to the contest lighter than the other competitors but well fuelled and rested.

The reward for doing this successfully is huge. Looking back at our example above it is definitely the case that a 75kg athlete has an advantage over a 68kg one with all else being equal – the larger athlete will be stronger, will hit harder and will usually be able to lift more weight; but the truth is that both of these individuals could compete in the 67.5kg class given water cutting and refuelling. If both manage to do it successfully, then even though both weighed the same amount at the time of testing, one will be significantly larger and at great advantage compared to the other. On the other hand a 7.5kg water cut for the heavier athlete, while possible, will involve some pretty serious interventions listed below and these could have a dramatically negative effect on performance, perhaps even health – a poorly timed cut or insufficient refuelling strategy could spell disaster.

Ultimately, effectively cutting weight is a skill. A skill that takes time, preparation, planning and understanding of not only safe water depletion strategies, but also an intelligent refuelling plan to rehydrate and restore full glycogen stores prior to the event. There are a number of techniques used, many of which will be listed below, some of which are easy, some are hard, some are safe and some (which we won't list in great detail) can be deadly – suffice it to say that a good coach and sensible competitor would never attempt an approach that they hadn't researched thoroughly and tested beforehand. Every fighter has his or her own way to lose the weight, some taking on board research driven methods, some still using dangerous methods that in the eyes of many should be banned from the sport.

Regardless of the techniques utilised there are numerous risks associated with losing large amounts of weight in a short amount of time through any methods involving water manipulation (which amounts to little more than planned dehydration). Some of these risks include poor performance, elevated heart rate, increased blood pressure, and higher risk of injury (14). Pair this with a hot day, a heavy bang to the head or lifting a heavy load and you can see how it can prove fatal for an individual who has not paid attention to their body (14). Cutting weight should never be attempted recklessly.

While water cutting is seen as part and parcel of professional sports, it is a concern to see it being so prevalent in amateur fighting and lifting. In these individuals, cutting weight becomes even more dangerous simply because unlike professional athletes, the level of education and sponsorship (including a dedicated team of nutritionists and other sports professionals) isn't as accessible to them. Amateur athletes are expected to make weight and compete within several hours of weigh ins. Due to the short amount of time between weigh in and competition, the fighters and lifters need to take every precaution they can to avoid cutting too much weight, for both health and performance reasons. Bouts or event weigh ins that are close to the event start allow very little time for re-fuelling strategies to take full effect and some athletes may go into an event dehydrated, under fuelled and at high risk of loss and injury. We will fully outline suggested approaches below.

26.6. Choosing a weight category

Choosing a weight category can be a daunting task. Most professionals will have spent years perfecting their sport and will understand where their strengths and weaknesses are, but most amateurs will be finding their feet and working through different weight categories to gauge how they feel and perform. Unfortunately finding your way around isn't the best method and there has to be some thought put into this process.

Even as a seasoned pro, moving up and down a weight class is risky – stepping down involves losing a lot of weight and often lean body mass, while stepping up a weight category means competing against people who are usually far ahead of you in terms of lean body mass and so you are at a disadvantage. That's why it's so impressive when some competitors manage to do it. If you're looking to jump up, it usually means a couple of frustrating years while you work to fill out your frame and adjust to the higher weight. Often the other problem is the one facing coaches, moving down a class.

One of the primary determinants for weight classes is height. This makes logical sense because most competitors in a given sport will have a roughly similar build, and so it is entirely expected that the heavier athletes will usually be taller (if the weight isn't coming from muscle or fat, it has to come from somewhere!). Of course there is variance and no two fighters or lifters will look the same or have the exact same physique, but it's rare to see two 80kg athletes in the same sport, one of which is a stocky 5ft 2 inches and the other a gangly 7ft tall.

For example, consider a 5ft, 11inches tall, 80kg (176lbs) male boxer who is holding a little too much bodyfat. Stepping in the ring at that weight would mean he would be fighting opponents of the same or similar weight, but who are at possibly 6ft and above with longer reaches, or who are far stronger than him due to weighing the same but having far more muscle mass. This could be a huge disadvantage because a taller opponent will have a greater punching/kicking range and be potentially faster and with greater endurance due to being leaner. The stronger opponent on the other hand may have greater endurance through virtue of carrying less fat weight but also more simply he's likely to hit harder. Therefore, it makes sense to bring our fighter down a weight category to welterweight.

Of course, getting down to that weight may make the athlete tired if not done efficiently, and he may perform at a lower threshold while feeling psychologically less confident. As such it's a really good idea to get your client to a beneficial bodyfat level which can be maintained year-round, before looking to start cutting weight in a more dramatic way. Remember, athletes water cut because they can't realistically cut more fat. If you have a lot of bodyfat to lose, look to address this first.

26.7. Choosing a weight category based on body fat level

In a weight class-based sport, being lean is important as it allows for maximum strength-to-weight ratio. Excess body fat is therefore problematic as it is taking up mass that could be replaced with muscle tissue at a given weight. Muscle has the obvious benefits of being able to generate power, provide strength and store glycogen and intramuscular triglycerides for immediate fuelling, so more muscle and less fat is good. However, it almost goes without saying that there is a cut-off point after which less fat is not a good thing. As with most things, there are problems at the extremes and there is a sweet-spot somewhere in the middle that we need to find. The exact bodyfat at which an athlete performs at their best will depend somewhat on their genetics, with many professional fighters showing up to bouts with differing bodyfat percentages, but that doesn't mean we can't make generalisations.

If the physiques of competitive athletes are anything to go by, between 6-13% bodyfat men seem to perform better (15). For some athletes the lower end may be ideal and for others they may do better at the top end or higher, for example 14-15% and a little higher is not uncommon in powerlifters, with many superheavyweight strength athletes carrying far more fat than this. A good approach is for athletes to look at the other competitors in their sport and try to achieve a similar level of conditioning. You need to work with your client to find a level of conditioning that lets them move well while also recovering and improving – essentially the focus should be on good nutrition, recovery and training optimally, with the weight the client lands at being taken as a good gauge of where they should be.

Whatever weight they achieve when they reach a bodyfat level comparative with other fighters, and a degree of fitness that leads you both to believe they are ready, can be considered a rough starting point for deciding on the weight class they will fall in to. Generally speaking, you'd look to meet the weight class below this weight unless the client is at the higher end of their bracket and already lean. If the athlete ends up very lean and fit at 74kg, it makes a lot of sense to hold this weight and compete in the 75kg class, but if they land at 70kg, a drop to the 67.5kg class is highly feasible. Experience comes in here, as does knowing the client well.

26.8. Losing weight

As we've discussed in detail, most athletes whose sport is weight related will tend to walk around at a higher weight than their fight weight, and we have mentioned the two means of actually bringing them down, namely cutting and losing weight. We will discuss the latter first because, it's the first one that you will actually do. Therefore, the first thing you need to do is decide what weight you are going to try to achieve.

We have already covered weight category band weights and what to do when a fighter or lifter is competing for the first time, but what if they have done it before? It is important to not just rely entirely on the weight the athlete last competed at. We need to take into consideration how they felt at that weight and how the competition went, how they have performed in training and what they had to do in order to reach the weight that they did (did they have to cut any weight?). We also have to think about how long ago it was, if the event was 6 years ago since last competing, it may be difficult to hit that weight again, maybe they have more muscle mass. This is where jumping up a weight category is an option. That being said, the vast majority of the time an athlete will compete in the same weight category competition to competition and so the first task is typically to help them drop some off-season fat mass, usually during a specified period of training known as meet prep for strength athletes or fight camp for fighters.

As you can imagine, this takes planning, and the more time you have with the athlete to work all this in, the better. The more fat mass the athlete has, the longer you will need to work with them because realistically it is a bad idea to lose a lot of weight during what will be a comparatively harder period of training that really tests the athlete's recovery. It's also not a good idea to take things all the way to the line, dieting right up until competition day. Bringing them close to their competition weight by the time you reach a few weeks out from the event allows you to practice depletion and refuelling strategies way before the event day; you don't want to be going in blind.

If you have an athlete hovering around 12-14% bodyfat 6 weeks out from an event, you have only 1-2kg to lose and a good time frame to plan out the weight cut and refuelling strategies. This is in contrast to other situations, for example if you had an athlete who was 20% bodyfat with 7-8kg to lose 8 weeks prior to an event, the process becomes far more difficult, and when you have 15kg to lose within the same timeframe it gets really complex. At this time you have to ask yourself a few questions:

- Could they move up a weight class?

- If they don't make weight, what will the penalty be?

- If they lose weight rapidly, is that going to really impact their sporting performance? (it probably will, but in sports like powerlifting you have more leeway than in sports like MMA, because the demands are different)

- How much do we think we can help them cut weight at the end of prep, ready for a weigh in?

- How much time will we have to refuel, and will that be enough?

We have to weigh up the odds, calculate the data and objectively assess what we have in front of us and make a tough decision. Generally speaking the recommendation for losing 0.5-1.5% of bodyweight per week applies here too, and so you can see that, for example, a client that weighs 80kg can lose roughly 0.4-1.2kg per week. Planning the timeframe of a weight drop in this manner is difficult because you don't know that the process will be linear (it often won't be) but it's effective enough to get some planning going. The end goal of the weight loss phase should be a fit, healthy and strong athlete who is within the 'error margin' listed below for different weight cutting times. Unless you have only 1-2 hours or so between weigh in and competition, you have time to refuel meaning you would be losing weight unnecessarily if you kept going until you reached the weight you had to be for your class. This risks excessive muscle loss, but it also risks becoming too lean and ending up fatigued.

Of course, this needs to be taken within the context noted above – most athletes walk around over competition weight. If a particular athlete simply stays 2-3kg overweight during the off-season then this can all be lost with no depletion needed. For the athlete walking around at 90kg and competing at 75kg, though, a combination of weight loss and weight cutting will be needed.

The remainder of the fat loss approach is no different to that mentioned earlier in this course – an adequate calorie deficit is important (though that needs to be carefully planned so as to manage performance during competition preparation), and macronutrients should be tailored towards the twin goals of maximal muscle retention and again, performance. Roughly 2.3-3.1g of protein per kilogram of lean body mass, less than 30% of dietary intake from fat and the remainder of calories coming from carbohydrate is the approach listed earlier in the course and is the one we recommend here. More information on this can be found in the fat loss programming and bodybuilding prep notes. The only thing of note here is that fat may need to reduce to 20% of intake in order to make sure carbohydrate intake is adequate for fuelling high levels of anaerobic activity in some athletes.

When you are planning the degree to which weight will be either lost or cut by your athlete, an important thing to keep in mind is the amount of time they have between being weighed and actually stepping into the ring or onto the platform, because it is that which largely dictates your approach.

26.9. Weigh-in times

Athletes will have somewhere between 1-36 hours between weigh-in and competition, with 4-24 hours being the norm. The only way to find out for your particular competition is to check the rules relevant to the federation or governing body. The days prior to the weigh in are referred to as the depletion phase, involving the gradual and deliberate dehydration of the client utilising a number of methods listed below. From the moment they step off the scale you are then in the replenishment stage where rehydrating and refuelling are the primary concern, to ensure the athlete is ready to go.

Clearly, those that have up to 36 hours from weigh-in to the event start time have plenty of room to work within their refuelling strategies, and it's not uncommon to see rapid weight loss in the form of weight cutting of more than 10% of their bodyweight leading up to the weigh-in (3). However, the recommendations for safe weight cutting strategies are closer to 2-5% of bodyweight (4), with the higher end being relevant to athletes with longer time and the lower end being shorter. Of course, you also need to take in to account the athlete's personal tolerance to weight cutting because while some athletes report being unaffected, others really struggle to compete having been dehydrated the day before. More on this in the section below.

This means that an athlete looking to compete at 75kg with a 36 hour weigh in, for example, could utilise weight loss until they were around 78-79kg then safely cut the rest. A little more would be possible but likely to cause decrements in performance and so would need to be tested beforehand. Conversely, if they had only 4 hours it would be wise to make sure they were roughly 76.5kg or less before undergoing the below depletion stage to cut water.

26.10. Depletion phase

The depletion phase is the time taken to acutely lose water and glycogen from the body.

The first and most obvious place to start is the simplest, glycogen depletion. The body holds 3g of water alongside each 1g of carbohydrates (5) in glycogen and with glycogen stores of between 400-500g being the average, this represents a significant opportunity for dropping weight. In fact, even at the low end of this range we have around 1.6kg that can be lost from this approach alone. It takes between 2-3 days of a Very Low Carbohydrate (VLC) environment to deplete glycogen stores in active people (6) meaning that it is also relatively easy to do this in the week or so prior to the competition. Many fighters opt to reduce their carbohydrate to ketogenic (or close to it) levels for the week before a competition, in the hopes of regaining their glycogen stores after weigh ins. A low fibre diet is also preferred as this reduces intestinal matter, thus aiding in further weight loss.

Perhaps the most common method of augmenting this weight loss is through manipulation of water, directly. Athletes will consume large amounts of water (one study on the topic used 100ml per kilogram of bodyweight (7)) roughly 7 days prior to competition, then decrease this significantly (the study mentioned dropped to 15ml per kilogram in the days before the fight). This approach seeks to dramatically increase urination by manipulating the rate at which the kidneys excrete water, then suddenly decrease it, leaving insufficient time for the kidneys to adapt before excess water (and thus weight) is lost. This is coupled with a normal salt intake, but sometimes with a very low one. This low salt approach (and in fact the practice in general) risks hyponatremia – an excessive and potentially harmful loss of blood electrolytes, but it is nonetheless effective (7) and one of the most common approaches to weight cutting (15).

However, this is not always as effective as the athlete would like and when they are a day out from competition they may find themselves to be still overweight. This is not an ideal scenario, and we may have to add in a few extra methods to push that last little bit of weight out as safely as possible. Hot baths, saunas, training in plastic suits and fasting are common practices which are comparatively safe provided the athlete pays close attention to how they are feeling and stops whatever they are doing as soon as they feel any negative symptoms. Beyond that there are natural diuretics that are utilised sometimes, alongside more dangerous and damaging (physically and mentally) approaches like laxatives, diet pills, strong diuretics and regular spitting (15). Needless to say, we do not endorse the latter list and will not discuss them further.

Looking back at the healthier options, there are a variety of ways to sweat water out including sitting in a hot sauna, hot tub, or bath tub. While they're all effective using a bath tub is generally the most commonly used as most people don't have access to a sauna or steam room. On top of that, a sauna comes with the added risk of making it very easy to overheat in general, and excessive sweating and heat can not only cause dehydration, but a loss of reported power and performance (10). Bathing could be considered safer. To use this approach:

- Fill the bathtub with hot water that's not too hot to cause harm. It obviously shouldn't be boiling but when you step inside, but it should be hotter than you'd ever consider bathing in (8)

- Slowly immerse as much of your body as possible in the water

- Soon as you start to sweat, stay in the bathtub for 10-20min then slowly get out for a break

- Dry yourself off and check your weight to see how much you lost in your first round. This will be a good gauge moving forward for the rest of the cut

- Repeat this process until you're roughly 0.5-1lb above what you need to weigh-in at. You'll lose the remainder of this the following day when you urinate/overnight in your breath

Things to think about when using a bath or sauna:

- If using one, make sure your bathtub doesn't have a limited supply of hot water because odds are, you're going to need to refill it several times. Hotel bath tubs tend to be fine, but some older homes and apartments don't have enough hot water to support a longer cut

- Keep as much of your body as possible (aside from your head) under water. If your arms and legs are hanging out above water, it'll take longer for your body to heat up and sweat

- Stay away from eating salty foods and drinking loads of water during the process. Sip a little if you need to in order to avoid extreme sensations of thirst, but realistically the point of this is to cause dehydration and so adding water back in is counterproductive

- You're going to be thirsty so bathing etc. should be done as close to the weigh in as possible so you don't have to suffer too long

- Don't take it too far. Remember, it's just an event. If you need to call it off and rehydrate in order to stay safe because you're feeling dizzy then your health is worth more than any competition. Next time spend more time losing weight or shift up a weight class. With that said if you are cutting a small amount of weight and paying attention to how you feel, you should be absolutely fine

As mentioned above a sweat suit is often used by competitors, too (15). This involves wearing a rubberised suit (often over the top of winter clothes) and either sitting in heat or exercising to cause huge amounts of sweating. This method can be very effective and some prefer it to bathing because of its efficacy, but it does result in the massive amounts of sweating we highlighted above as being potentially damaging to overall performance. As such this should be seen as a real last resort, and again it cannot be stressed enough that an athlete electing to cut weight in this manner must pay extremely close attention to how they feel, and cease all activity if dizziness occurs.

Dandelion root is a popular herb for use during weight cutting. Dandelion is used for many conditions, but so far there isn't enough scientific evidence to determine whether or not it is effective for any of them. However there is some empirical data that suggests dandelion root can act as a mild diuretic to increase urination (9). It must be noted that diuretics are banned by the IOC, and some federations include dandelion in with that, so you need to be careful. Stronger diuretics are extremely dangerous, and we do not condone their usage under any non-medical circumstances.

Another interesting avenue to consider is an athlete's creatine supplementation – perhaps the most popular non-stimulant ergogenic aid there is. Creatine supplementation causes water retention because it's stored as creatine phosphate alongside water within muscle cells (11). A decision must be made therefore, as to whether the athlete wants to lose the 1-2kg they may lose by ceasing supplementation or whether they want to maintain the small performance benefit. Ultimately, this decision is up to the athlete, though it's worth considering that a small percentage reduction in performance is a trivial price to pay for an acute form of weight loss that doesn't involve dehydration via the methods mentioned above.

If any method beyond glycogen depletion is used (realistically this will have to happen unless the weigh in is 24 hours or longer) then it needs to be appreciated that if there is one thing your body hates, it's being dehydrated. Everything stops functioning the way it should and you become tired, weak, and lack co-ordination, three things that you need functioning to stay on top of your game. Even performing seemingly simple tasks like thinking and reacting at speed are impaired when only 2% dehydrated (12) and so fighters have to make sure they know exactly how much weight they can cut and put back on to ensure an optimal performance. When weight cuts are taken to extremes, performance is impaired and the risk of injury is increased. (13).

The first thing to do is find out how long you have to refeed and rehydrate after the weigh in. If a weigh in is 24 hours you should have no problem using all of the methods listed above (to a degree relative to athlete tolerance) because refuelling is relatively simple over 24 hours. If, however, the weigh in is only a short amount of time (say 4 hours) before the competition then you will need to assess your options carefully. The athlete is not going to be able to rapidly replenish glycogen stores fully within that time because 400g or so of carbohydrate will take a long time to digest even when using the rapidly absorbed liquid carbohydrate solutions discussed below. As such a short time necessitates modest carbohydrate and water manipulation in tandem, whereas longer timeframes allow for carbohydrate restriction to do more of the 'heavy lifting' as well as affording a longer time to rehydrate fully.

Overall, with short weigh in times the goal should be to lose weight as close to the relevant category as possible, cutting as little as you realistically can. The risk just isn't worth it.

Below is a real world example of what a weight cut could look like, using BTN Academy tutor Simon Herbert's 4kg cut. As you can see, the majority of the difference comes from modest carbohydrate manipulation and some fluctuation in water, rather than anything dramatic – the key thing is not to see who can cut the most weight, but who can win on the day!

Simon Herbert fight peak week example

Peak week starts Saturday dropping from 450g of carbohydrates to 350g, protein and fats stay the same, water is relatively high at 4 litres. Only slight adjustments in carbohydrate and water manipulation were made in the last week up to weigh-in.

Fig. 84

Day	Protein	Carbs	Fat	Body mass (kg)	Water intake and sodium
Saturday	185	350	80	82	4ltr normal water normal sodium
Sunday	185	350	80		4ltr normal water normal sodium
Monday	185	350	80		4ltr normal water normal sodium
Tuesday	185	350	80		3ltr water normal sodium
Wednesday Stop training	185	250	80	81.2	2ltr water normal sodium
Thursday Walk	185	-150g	80		1.5ltr water normal sodium
Friday-rest	185	-150g	80	80	1ltr water normal sodium

A hot bath was needed to reduce weight from 78.6kg at 10am down to the goal weight of 78kg, then once that was done it was time to refuel and rehydrate over the next 36 hours.

Fig. 85

Weigh-in day			
	6am	12pm/weigh-in Weighed in at 78kg	Immediately post-weigh-in
Macros	P20, F5, C0	-	P30, C>100, F10
Water	Sip	Sip	Large bolus, then as required

26.11. Refuelling and hydration strategies

The purpose of the refuelling stage is not necessarily to gain weight per se (though this will happen) but to regain lost glycogen and water in order to be properly fuelled and hydrated for competition.

Carbohydrates are perhaps the easiest thing to refuel with. After a depletion phase, 8-10g/kg/bw of bodyweight has been shown to increase performance in endurance athletes by super-compensating glycogen stores (15), and so this is the level that is recommended if total glycogen depletion has been used. Of course, for lesser carbohydrate restriction, consuming roughly 150% of the athlete's typical carbohydrate intake during the hours before the competition is a reasonable approach. Needless to say, these carbohydrates will likely be high GI because this reduces gastric upset, especially if the weigh in is a short time before the actual event. In fact, as you have learned the rate at which carbohydrate can be absorbed into the blood is limited by the rate at which it can leave the small intestine, and it does so via transporter proteins.

Two different transporter proteins are utilised to help carbohydrates leave the small intestine – GLUT-5 used by fructose, and a sodium-dependent glucose transporter known as SGLT-1 which transports glucose and galactose. Saturation of the SGLT transporter can limit glucose transport and so consuming carbohydrates from multiple sources can increase the rate at which carbohydrates are absorbed into the blood (16). As such, consuming a fructose/glucose drink would be a great way to kickstart the recovery process more efficiently than glucose alone, and if that drink is 6-10% glucose this could also assist with retaining water (17).

This will also help with retaining water. If you have used only carbohydrate cutting to induce weight loss this will be less important – simply return your client to their usual water intake, plus some more, in order to replenish glycogen, drinking to thirst beyond this point. If dehydration is used, it's very important to take note of how much weight is lost. After dehydration your client will need to consume roughly 150% of their lost weight (expressed as 1 litre per kg lost) (17), ideally in a hypotonic solution, such as diluted Lucozade (14). Adding 5-10g of creatine to this mixture will help restore hydration levels too (14).

This mixture should be consumed over a number of hours. Consuming all of it in one sitting results in a greater amount of urination than does consuming it over a prolonged period (17), so it would not be a good idea to drink 1-2 litres of water in the space of an hour or two. Again this further illustrates that cutting more than 2% of the client's bodyweight from a combination of carbohydrate and water restriction is a bad idea when the weigh in time is close to competition.

To wrap up, the client should start their replenishment period by consuming a drink containing an amount of liquid representing a sizeable proportion of the athlete's lost weight, expressed as litres per kilogram. However, not all of their lost weight (unless this is a small amount) as their total rehydration needs to be spread out. This would ideally be hypotonic in terms of electrolytes, meaning diluted isotonic beverages or something else with roughly 50-100mg of sodium per 100ml (17). If the client needs to replenish glycogen rapidly, this drink should also be 10% carbohydrate by weight, or potentially higher if time is of the essence. Do test this, as the client's tolerance to carbohydrate bolus dosing may vary. Adding some creatine is a good idea as it promotes further muscle hydration.

After this meals should be chosen based on a high carbohydrate content (from low GI sources) with a moderate sodium content to promote further water storage. Protein and fat are important but must be considered afterthoughts – sushi is a popular option for this time, for a reason.

26.12. Summary and off-season weight

You have heard this point numerous times up until now, the more weight the client has to lose, the higher chance of performance impairment there is leading up to a competition (as well as muscle loss if the client is losing fat, too). Therefore, we want to devise a plan that allows the athlete to be within 6-8kg of their fight weight in the off-season, or where they feel their best in training. A weight drop that is manageable based on their weight category, is a much safer way of bringing the athlete closer to a win. There may be times where there are multiple weight categories to hit over the year. This entails further planning and potentially the choice to have to say no to some events if the process is unsafe, unethical and doesn't fit in with the long-term plan. Working alongside their strength coaches, physios, and other professional team players (if they have one) allows you to understand the plans that have been laid out, the course of action to take and essentially to be part of a team that has the athlete's best interests and safety at heart. Weight cutting is effective and when done right can lead to a significant advantage (or at least the avoidance of a disadvantage if the opponent(s) do(es) it too but doing it wrong could spell disaster. Remember, the dose makes the poison, and there's a big difference between 2kg of dehydration and 8kg.

26.13. References

1. AIBA, Technical & Competition Rules, §1.2 & Appendix K.

2. Usapowerlifting.com. (2018). [online] Available at: http://www.usapowerlifting.com/wp-content/uploads/2014/01/USAPL-Rulebook-2017.pdf [Accessed 29 May 2018].4.

3. Franchini, E., Brito, C. and Artioli, G. (2012). Weight loss in combat sports: physiological, psychological and performance effects. Journal of the International Society of Sports Nutrition, 9(1), p.52.

4. Artioli GG, Gualano B, Franchini E, Scagliusi FB, Takesian M, Fuchs M, Lancha AH: Prevalence, magnitude, and methods of rapid weight loss among judo competitors. Med Sci Sports Exerc. 2010, 42: 436-442.

5. Fernández-Elías, V., Ortega, J., Nelson, R. and Mora-Rodriguez, R. (2015). Relationship between muscle water and glycogen recovery after prolonged exercise in the heat in humans. European Journal of Applied Physiology, 115(9), pp.1919-1926.

6. Acheson, K., Schutz, Y., Bessard, T., Anantharaman, K., Flatt, J. and Jéquier, E. (1988). Glycogen storage capacity and de novo lipogenesis during massive carbohydrate overfeeding in man. The American Journal of Clinical Nutrition, 48(2), pp.240-247.

7. Reale, R., Slater, G., Cox, G., Dunican, I. and Burke, L. (2018). The Effect of Water Loading on Acute Weight Loss Following Fluid Restriction in Combat Sports Athletes. International Journal of Sport Nutrition and Exercise Metabolism, pp.1-9.

8. Reale, R., Slater, G. and Burke, L. (2017). Acute-Weight-Loss Strategies for Combat Sports and Applications to Olympic Success. International Journal of Sports Physiology and Performance, 12(2), pp.142-151.

9. Clare, B., Conroy, R. and Spelman, K. (2009). The Diuretic Effect in Human Subjects of an Extract ofTaraxacum officinaleFolium over a Single Day. The Journal of Alternative and Complementary Medicine, 15(8), pp.929-934.

10. Gutierrez, A., Mesa, J., Chirosa, J. and Castillo, M. (2003). Sauna-Induced Rapid Weight Loss Decreases Explosive Power in Women but not in Men. International Journal of Sports Medicine, 24(7), pp.518-522.

11. Powers, M., Arnold, B., Weltman, A., Perrin, D., Mistry, D., Kahler, D., Kraemer, W. and Volek, J. (2003). Creatine Supplementation Increases Total Body Water Without Altering Fluid Distribution. Journal of Athletic Training, 38(1), pp.44-50.

12. Barr, S. (1999). Effects of Dehydration on Exercise Performance. Canadian Journal of Applied Physiology, 24(2), pp.164-172.

13. Franchini, E., Brito, C. and Artioli, G. (2012). Weight loss in combat sports: physiological, psychological and performance effects. Journal of the International Society of Sports Nutrition, 9(1), p.52.

14. Puttuck, L. and Palmieri, M. (2014). Correlation between body composition and biomechanical measurements of performance for mixed martial arts athletes – a pilot study. Journal of the International Society of Sports Nutrition, 11(Suppl 1), p.P28.

15. Giannini Artioli, G., Gualano, B., Franchini, E., Scagliusi, F., Takesian, M., Fuchs, M. And Lancha, A. (2010). Prevalence, Magnitude, and Methods of Rapid Weight Loss among Judo Competitors. Medicine & Science in Sports & Exercise, 42(3), pp.436-442.

16. Jentjens, R.L., L. Moseley, R.H. Waring, L.K. Harding, and A.E. Jeukendrup (2004a). Oxidation of combined ingestion of glucose and fructose during exercise. J. Appl. Physiol. 96: 1277-1284.

17. Evans, G., James, L., Shirreffs, S. and Maughan, R. (2017). Optimizing the restoration and maintenance of fluid balance after exercise-induced dehydration. Journal of Applied Physiology, 122(4), pp.945-951.